Be a Surviv

Lung Cancer Treatment Guide

Third Edition

VLADIMIR LANGE, MD

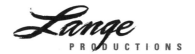

Lange
PRODUCTIONS

Dedicated to
cancer survivors
everywhere

Table of Contents

Our Consultants

**This book was developed with the invaluable assistance
of the following leading experts:**

Pamela Matten, RN, BSN, OCN, Editor

Terri Ades, PhD, FNP-BC, AOCN
Behnam Ebrahimi, MD
Mark R. Huber, MD
Edward Levitt, Survivor and Advocate
Barbara Rabinowitz, PhD, LCSW, RN
Swapnil Rajurkar, MD
Juliann Reiland-Smith, MD
Kathleen L. Schneekloth, MD
Kimberly Stump-Sutliff, RN, MSN, AOCNS
Ivy C. Tuason, RN, MSN, FNP
Benny Weksler, MD
Kathy Yeatman-Stock, LCSW

Special thanks to:

Pomona Valley Hospital Medical Center, Lung Cancer Program
St. Joseph Hospital of Orange, Thoracic Oncology Program
for on-location photography at their beautiful facilities.

Sincere gratitude to:
Johnson Lightfoote, MD for the use of his outstanding images.

THANK YOU...

...to the survivors and their loved ones for sharing their stories.
Your insight will enlighten, and your words will inspire,
those who follow you on this journey.

Ali Desiderio

Lou Gideon

Tomma Hargraves

Richard Hergenrather, PhD

Stephanie Hineline

Edward Levitt

Linda Levitt

Kay Scholtz

Mary Ann Volpe

Wells Whitney

ACKNOWLEDGMENTS

No single physician or author can do justice to a topic as complex as lung cancer. I have been fortunate to have had the help and support of many knowledgeable colleagues. It is their guidance and expertise that make this book a balanced, informative and accurate tool that will help you deal with your disease.

I also want to thank the survivors and their partners who candidly shared their stories. This book has been greatly enriched by your contributions.

Finally, all of us who worked on this book want to thank the patients—the ones from whom we learn so much and the ones who contribute to research studies that allow us to advance the treatment and understanding of the disease. This book is for you, and for those who will follow in your footsteps to recovery.

INTRODUCTION TO THE THIRD EDITION

The last edition of this book was about empowerment. About making you feel strong and informed enough to take an active participation in your treatment and recovery. For this edition I must add "hope" as a new theme. Because dramatic changes in treatment options introduced in the past few years greatly increase your opportunities for successful outcomes.

Perhaps the only thing worse than being handed a diagnosis of lung cancer, is the feeling of confusion that follows. You may be overwhelmed by the torrent of information that is coming at you. You may feel unable to understand why certain treatments are being recommended. You don't seem to have enough facts to make the decisions you are being asked to make. And you may feel like a pawn in a game being played by strangers.

I have experienced these feelings personally. Many years ago my wife was diagnosed with breast cancer. Even though both of us are physicians, we understood little, and remembered even less, of the new and complex information that was thrown at us during our initial meeting with the doctors. It was weeks before we were able to unravel all the details, and begin deciding on a course of treatment. Those were weeks of feeling completely disempowered.

That confusion lead me to create the *Be a Survivor* series of cancer treatment guides. Several features make the *Be a Survivor Lung Cancer Treatment Guide* different from other books on the topic:

The explanations are in simple and clear terms, and are illustrated with helpful diagrams and photographs—a style that makes the information suitable to all readers.

To make the information as balanced and objective as possible, I worked closely with a wide variety of medical experts in each field of cancer treatment. This means that the book is truly multidisciplinary, rather than biased toward a single specialist's point of view.

I enhanced the book with candid comments by patients and their partners —the women and men who "have been there" and whose stories will help you understand better your own feelings and challenges at this difficult time. Their voices will inspire and empower you.

As I began writing this book, I was surprised by how few lung cancer books are available. And I was stunned by their lack of a positive outlook.

This book was written to send you a message of hope. Today, lung cancer is not the automatic death sentence it once was. New technologies and new medications are being introduced every day. So as you go through the treatment process, always keep in mind that today you have the best chance ever to be a survivor.

How to Use This Book

I organized the book in a way that mirrors your path through treatment and recovery.

First, I've offered a few suggestions on how to cope with the feelings you might experience after you learn that you have lung cancer. Facing the disease with as clear a head as possible will help you make the right decisions.

Next, I listed a few tips on how to assemble a team of skilled healthcare providers to ensure that you get the best care possible, and surround yourself with a network of caring supporters to help you get through the tough times. Think of it as building a safety net.

I also included information on complementary treatments, such as meditation, acupuncture, and spiritual support. Many people find these to be valuable additions to their battle with cancer.

One of the last chapters of the book offers suggestions on how you can make a smooth transition from treatment to recovery, both emotionally and physically. It also tells you how to follow-up with your doctor, and how to keep yourself as healthy as possible.

There is a chapter written for your partner - husband, wife, or special person in your life. The information will help this person to be the best supporter for you, without neglecting his or her own needs.

And there is a chapter that addresses the issues that may surface if the treatments fail to achieve their goal.

Each chapter includes lists of questions that you might want to address to your healthcare professionals. For your convenience, these questions are repeated at the end of the book, on sheets that you can tear out. Take these sheets with you on office visits, to help you communicate more effectively with your physicians and nurses.

Use this book as a guide to help you understand all aspects of your treatment and recovery, so that you can become an active partner with your medical team.

I, and the many dedicated healthcare professionals who worked with me on this book, wish you a speedy recovery.

CHAPTER 1

FACING LUNG CANCER

COPING STRATEGIES

"You have lung cancer." These may be the most frightening words you've ever heard. You may feel scared, angry, crushed—or you may be in complete denial. And for good reason. Lung cancer has a reputation for being difficult, if not impossible, to treat.

First of all, you need to know that a diagnosis of lung cancer is not an automatic death sentence. Medical science is making new strides every day and finding better ways to deal with this challenging disease.

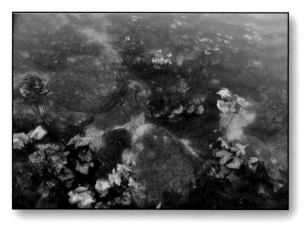

What *is* a death sentence is to give up without a fight. The best approach you can take is to resolve, right now, that you will do everything you can to make sure your treatment is successful. Tell yourself that losing this battle is simply not an option. This positive attitude may be your best ally through the tough times that may come.

ED: The doctor was like a mortician: "Here is the news. You have cancer. All over your body. There is nothing I can offer you. You should go home and make your... arrangements," he told me. "You have about eight months."

But he had the wrong guy. I am a proactive fellow. I said, "Screw this!" That very day I resigned from the company I was running, and set out to fight my lung cancer.

That was eleven years ago.

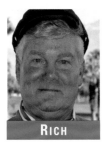

RICH

I've always been athletic, I never smoked – where was this coming from? I thought, now what? I have a family to care for, I have work to do. And my bucket list? I already ran a marathon, and I got a PhD, but I didn't climb Everest yet! So, you know… I have to keep going!

So, where do you begin?

I have listed some of the first steps that you need to take to help you process through your feelings and fears. Take a few minutes to understand them, and to decide how you want to proceed.

> • Acknowledge your feelings, realize that they are normal, but don't let them affect your judgement.
>
> • Assemble a team of healthcare professionals, friends and peers to help you. You cannot and should not face cancer alone.
>
> • Learn all you can about the disease and the different treatment options that are available.
>
> • Most importantly, become an active participant in your treatment and recovery.

UNDERSTANDING YOUR FEELINGS

The first few weeks after your diagnosis may be the hardest to handle. You may spend hours dwelling on questions such as "Why me?" or "Will the cancer kill me?" Or you might find yourself feeling "blue" and depressed to the point of not caring about the outcome of your disease. You might snap in anger or frustration at friends and at loved ones.

This confusing roller coaster of emotions is normal. Don't be too hard on yourself if your emotions slip out of your control every once in a while. You are going through a lot, and you don't need to be in perfect balance all of the time.

If you cannot deal with your feelings on your own, look for help. The best thing to do is to find someone you can talk to about what you are experiencing. This should be a mature, well-adjusted person who can listen with-

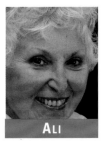

ALI

I had a CT scan to figure out why my stomach was hurting. They called with "good news, bad news." Stomach was fine, but I had a mass on my lung. That scan saved my life.

out passing judgment. Very close friends or family members may not be the best choice, because they can be too involved in the situation to remain objective.

Ask your doctor, nurse, or social worker for a referral to a professional counselor, or to a local support group of cancer survivors who meet regularly to offer mutual support and encouragement.

Psychiatrists, psychologists, and social workers can be very helpful with problems such as depression, panic attacks, feelings of isolation, anger, and other issues that may concern you.

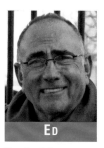

ED

I'm healthy as an ox. I run stairs, I work out. The only reason I went to see a doctor is because a pain in my leg interfered with my kickboxing. They found a lesion in my bone. And then one in my lungs.

ED: The doc said, "There is nothing I can do for you." It was a blow. My wife and I had worked so hard, planning for the future, for our retirement. For the first time since my father died, I cried.

After we left the doctor's office, my wife and I went home to make funeral arrangements. I helped her make them. The only thing I could not bring myself to do was choose a coffin. Just couldn't. I told her to just pick the cheapest pine box. Who wants to be remembered by the pretty brass handles, anyway?

DEALING WITH GUILT

In most peoples' minds, lung cancer is linked to smoking. So if you are, or were, a smoker, it is natural that one of the first thoughts to leap into your mind is, "I brought this on myself. Oh, why did I smoke?!" The guilt and regret you may be feeling may be even worse than the fear of the cancer itself.

Let me tell you about a very sophisticated medical device, often used by both physicians and laymen. It is called the *retrospectoscope*. It consists of two parts. A rear view mirror, for close examination of things you didn't do, and a whip, for repeatedly punishing yourself for not having done them.

QUESTIONS TO ASK YOUR COUNSELOR:

- **How do other people deal with this diagnosis?**

- **How do I get rid of the guilt I feel about smoking?**

- **How can I help my loved ones handle their feelings about my diagnosis?**

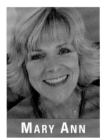

MARY ANN

Somehow people feel like you did it to yourself, even if you never smoked. Don't let that affect you. Who cares what those people think! Yes, I smoked. But I decided I couldn't go on kicking myself for it. It was over and done. Time to concentrate on dealing with my cancer.

ED

We started our own group in Georgia. When they come to me and say, "I am dying," I say, "Don't give me that crap!" I don't do compassion. You want compassion, talk to my wife.

Put the retrospectoscope down! Instead of driving with eyes glued to the past, focus on what lies ahead. Do the best you can with the cards you have been dealt.

Some lung cancer patients find comfort in the fact that two out of ten lung cancers occur in people who never even touched a cigarette. Others dwell on the statistic that the vast majority of smokers live to a ripe old age without ever having any respiratory problems. Use whatever thinking will allow you to feel better about the smoking, and move forward. Now is not the time to feel guilty. Now is the time to make changes that will have a positive effect on your life.

And, by the way, it's never too late to quit smoking. It will do wonders in helping you get through the treatment, particularly surgery and its side effects. So, put the cigarette down, too.

If you never smoked, or stopped a long time ago, you may be inclined to place blame on those responsible for generating second hand smoke. Or you may wonder if you had been exposed to something harmful at work, or in the environment. More than likely, you will never know what caused your lung cancer. Right now, how or why you wound up with lung cancer is not nearly as important as what you do next.

ED: There is definitely a stigma to lung cancer. People have the attitude that you brought it on yourself. And nobody supports us. Nobody is running around with pink ribbons.

Bottom line, makes no difference why you got it. Does it make any difference why you got hit by a truck? Just get up and fix it!

DEALING WITH THE FEAR OF DYING

When you are told you have lung cancer, it is perfectly normal to think about long-term outcomes and death. The thought of dying may also be unavoidable during certain times of your treatment.

Don't let these thoughts paralyze you or prevent you from putting up the best fight you can. If you say to yourself, "What is the use? Most of the patients with this condition will die anyway," you will be signing your own death warrant. Don't do it. If you find yourself losing hope, find someone —or something—to give you that proverbial "kick in the pants."

If your diagnosis has been handed to you just a few days ago, you need to take one step at a time. This is not the time to dwell on lung cancer mortality figures. Your energy should be focused on learning everything you can about your disease. And I mean about *your* disease, not about what happens to other people with other types of lung cancer.

Become an active participant and work with your healthcare team. Try to get an idea of what lies ahead. Do not dwell on the *worst* possible outcome, but strive to achieve the *best* possible outcome.

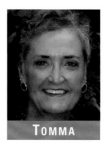

TOMMA

I had done all the right things. I stopped smoking 23 years ago. I ate right. I exercised a ton. And yet, there it was. A little nodule on the side of the neck. I said, this can't be right.

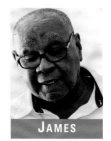

JAMES

My cancer was Stage 3B. All the way into the lymph nodes. Scary doesn't begin to describe it. So I prayed to die with dignity. But maybe even to survive.

STEPHANIE: At the time I was diagnosed with the lung and the breast cancers, my husband was dying of bladder cancer. So my first taught was, Oh my God, what is going to happen to my daughter? My eight-year-old is going to wind up an orphan!

But I have a strong faith. And I thought that it couldn't be God's will that both my husband and I die. I had to survive. For my daughter. I wasn't going down without a fight!

"DOCTOR, WHAT IS MY PROGNOSIS?"

Many patients want to know what they can expect so that they can prepare for the future – physically, financially, logistically and emotionally.

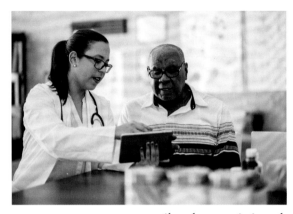

You may have seen the statistics for lung cancer survival – "X-percent will survive for X-many years." At first glance, the numbers are not encouraging. Try not to focus on the statistics for death from lung cancer. You are an individual, not a statistic. Your experience may be very different from others you have heard about.

It may be helpful to understand why general survival statistics may or may not apply to you. Survival statistics average out the number of patients with similar characteristics who lived for five years after being diagnosed. Notice the word "average". The numbers don't tell you the expected survival time for a specific individual. Yours may be much longer.

ALI: I took the plunge and asked my oncologist what my chances were. He got kind of serious. "50-50?" I asked. He shook his head. "Worse? 30-70?" "More like 15% chance you'll survive." I never won the lottery, and my divorce settlement sucked. So I figured it was my turn to be a winner. I decided I was going to be in the 15% who were going to make it.

In addition, a "five-year survival" reflects the result achieved with a method or drug that is at least five years old. It doesn't take into account the newer, more effective treatment options available today.

LINDA - Ed's Wife: They wanted to give Ed a drug that is used strictly to help the radiation. And... surprise!! The tumor shrunk 70% almost immediately, just from the drug, not from the radiation. The unexpected happens. You really need to find a doc who will think out of the box.

SHARING THE NEWS

Communicating With Your Partner

Try to remember that your spouse or life partner may be affected by your diagnosis as much as you are. It is best to involve her or him as soon as possible, so the two of you can find strength in each other, and learn from the beginning how you can work as a team.

In some ways the spouse's or partner's challenge may be particularly difficult because he will have to manage his own emotions, and at the same time shoulder the task of being your key supporter.

The key to protecting and preserving your relationship during these challenging times is communication. Honest, open conversations are often difficult and painful, but they are necessary.

Telling Your Family

The people who are close to you also will be affected by your news. They too may need to be angry, cry, and express their emotions. It's a natural part of adjusting to your diagnosis. It will help both you and your loved ones to talk openly about each other's feelings.

You may want to open the discussion yourself by asking them how they are doing with your diagnosis. This gives them a chance to voice what they are going through. It also shows them that you know – and care – that your diagnosis affects them as well. But be sure that you are ready to hear their fears before posing the questions. Pick a time when you feel strong and confident enough to be supportive of them.

Open communication from the start will go a long way toward strengthening the bonds with your loved ones, and securing the support you'll need.

LINDA - Ed's Wife - 15 years later: It has been a long and difficult journey. He is doing great and his attitude and willingness to live on never waivers. The immunotherapy is buying precious time.

ALI

The news was overwhelming, but I kept it to myself for a few days, because I didn't want to ruin my family's Easter holiday.

QUESTIONS TO ASK
YOUR DOCTOR:

- **Can I bring members of my family, or a friend, to talk to you directly?**

- **What should I tell my loved ones about my condition?**

- **Can you refer me to a counselor or to a support group specializing in lung cancer?**

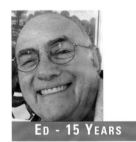

ED - 15 YEARS

I survived lung cancer, and brain metastases and abdominal metastases. But I still walk, although now I need a cane. No big deal. The point is, I am beating the odds.

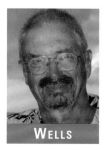

WELLS

Be proactive. Reach out.
Reach out to friends, to colleagues. There is nothing
sadder than someone who
shrinks into himself. Find
yourself one person who will
become your sounding board.

Dealing With Friends And Others

Friends can be an excellent source of help and support, particularly if you keep them informed, and let them help you.

Most will want to help, but may be unsure of how to go about it, and may be waiting for clues from you about where to begin. Make specific requests for simple things—to run an errand, prepare a meal, come for a visit. These small acts bring friends back into contact and help them feel useful and needed.

Bear in mind that most people have no experience dealing with cancer, and no idea what is expected or acceptable. "Isn't it too personal to ask about his surgery?" or "Should I pretend nothing happened?" or "How do I discuss his fears with him, without making things worse?" Help them by being the first to bring up whatever subject you want to discuss.

Sometimes the best friends seem to abandon you. Often this is their way of avoiding coming face-to-face with their own mortality. Don't take their perceived withdrawal personally, and don't hesitate to be the first to reach out and bring them back.

On the other hand, you may find that the interest is too intrusive. This is more likely to be the case in the beginning, when your diagnosis is "news" and your entire extended circle of friends wants to check in and see how you are doing.

Don't feel obligated to share all the details just because someone asks. It is okay to say, "Thanks for asking, but today I'd prefer to talk about something else."

If you are fortunate to have more than a handful of friends and acquaintances, this surge in interest may result in the phone ringing off the hook 24/7.

You may want to delegate the task of running the information center to one person, whose job will be to shield you from unwanted excesses in well-wishing. Empower that person to "just say no" to callers.

RICH

The thing that you must do
is stay positive. Be around
people who are positive. Get
involved in others' lives.
Turn around and help them
instead. That's how you get
through this ordeal.

ASSEMBLING YOUR SUPPORT NETWORK

One of your first steps after you hear your diagnosis should be to establish a network of people who can help you. This network will include your loved ones, your peer support groups, and of course a solid team of health-care professionals.

Friends and Family

In most cases your loved ones will provide the emotional support and closeness you need. They will also help you sort out facts and fears.

Try to select one person—your spouse, your partner, or best friend—who will accompany you when you meet with your physicians, or go to your treatments.

This companion can help you ask questions, remember information, or write down instructions. He can also serve as the clearing house for the volumes of information that your friends will collect from the internet and bring to your attention.

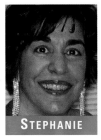

STEPHANIE

People want to help. But you have to tell them what you need. I would just ask, Can you order my Netflix? Can you cook me dinner? Can you help with the laundry? People just need suggestions.

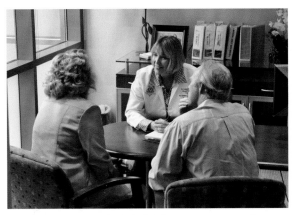

A companion can be helpful during your consultations.

He can become the center of your support network, acting as your sounding board, helping you to make decisions, coordinating support from friends and family, and at times shielding you from excessive attention.

STEPHANIE: I am blessed with a great support circle. My colleagues donated 300 work days so I could take all the time I needed to have my treatments. My friends chipped in to hire me a housekeeper. It was great to be able to devote all my energy to recovering.

Support Groups

Consider joining a support group. Support groups are groups of people who meet regularly, under the guidance of a trained facilitator, to discuss the participants' concerns.

Programs are organized in a variety of ways. Some groups meet only a few times; others are long-term, enabling members to work through problems. Some are composed of people with the same disease (for example, breast or colon cancer patients), others are selected by age or background. Some are just for patients; others include family or other special people.

Support groups give you a chance to openly discuss your thoughts with others who are going through the same experience. Meet other survivors who may be just a step or two ahead of you in their treatment, who can give you the hope you need to get through the challenges of your own treatment. Many hospitals consider some form of group counseling to be a necessary part of the standard treatment.

Visit the support group you are considering a couple of times before joining, so you can be sure that the peer mix meets your needs and expectations.

If you are unable to get out of the house, or live too far from the meeting location, you may choose to join an on-line support group.

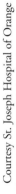

Courtesy St. Joseph Hospital of Orange

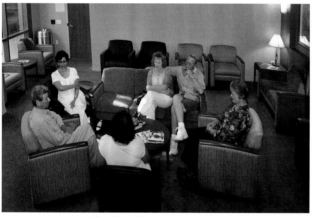

Support groups offer friendly settings to discuss your concerns.

ALI: I am not much of a support group person. And I don't do shrinks. But in The Wellness Community I found all the support I needed. I've met my match.

PARTNERING WITH YOUR HEALTHCARE TEAM

Cancer is a complicated disease and no single physician can be an expert in all aspects of the treatment you may need. Developing a treatment plan is a complex task that will involve a number of healthcare professionals—a real team of experts—who will give you their recommendations.

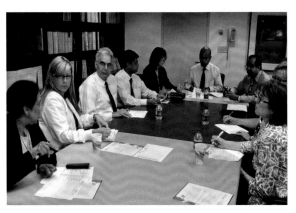

Some hospitals and cancer centers already have such teams of experts, called *multidisciplinary* teams. If your hospital doesn't, the National Cancer Institute or the American Cancer Society have resources to help you find healthcare professionals to add to your team.

Working as a team, medical experts can develop a better treatment plan for you.

Asking Questions

OK, let's be honest. There *is* such a thing as a stupid question. But *not* when it comes to cancer, and especially your lung cancer. Ask away. In this book, every chapter has a list of questions to ask your provider. Use these lists as a starting point to create your own questions about issues that are most important to you personally. Bring the lists to your medical meetings, and don't stop asking until all your questions have been answered to your satisfaction.

You may find that you need medical words defined, pictures drawn, or pamphlets or DVDs to take home. Enlist the help of a friend or relative who might be more science-savvy than you to help you process all the information that is likely to be given to you in the beginning.

WELLS: Get yourself a team of doctors. Make sure they work together and with you. The first one I picked was a young, aggressive, innovative guy. Gradually I acquired a bunch of doctors. When I came to a critical turning point in my treatment, I would survey all my doctors. "What do you think? How about you, what do you think?"

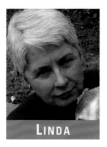

LINDA

If a doctor tells me there is
nothing he can do, he is not
the doctor I want. You really
can't go with the first guy
you see because he is more
convenient, or because you
like him. You need a real
cancer center, with doctors
that give you hope.

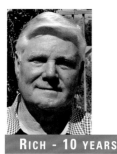

RICH - 10 YEARS

As I look back, it is amazing
how fast they acted. One day
I was fine, three days later I
had surgery. I sort of wish I
had time to evaluate my
options.

Getting A Second Opinion

Selecting the right course of treatment for your cancer is probably the most important decision you will ever face. For your own peace of mind, now and in the future, get a "second opinion"—an evaluation of your case by another physician, or a team of specialists. Consider getting even a third one. An amazing number of patients report getting a different assessment of their disease and treatment plans from their second set of medical consultants.

Keep in mind that most physicians will tend to offer you only the therapies that are available at their facilities. So take the time to "shop around". Go outside of your healthcare network, or outside your doctor's immediate community, away from any local medical politics, to be sure your case is viewed with a fresh perspective.

For you, a second opinion may be one of the most valuable and reassuring pieces of information. Get one. Remember, it is your body. You are entitled to evaluate all your options, and no competent healthcare provider will object if you seek another viewpoint. If nothing else, it will help you go forward with your treatment without second-guessing your choice.

Do ask your insurance company about their policy on second opinions. Some insist on it, some do not pay for it.

WELLS: The critical decision was to not accept my surgeon's thinking that I was not a surgical candidate. I said, "Chemo shrunk my tumor. Take a chance on me. Take my tumor out." I knew I would still have small tumors left, but I would figure out how to deal with them. I am not cured, I live with my lung cancer like a chronic disease. But I am alive!

Changing Doctors

Sometimes you may find that you are not getting along with one of the physicians treating you. The physician may seem abrupt, aloof, and uncaring, or fails to convince you of his competence. If this creates a barrier, let the physician know you wish to see someone else. The physician is probably as aware as you that a good relationship has not been established, and will be happy to transfer your records to another practitioner.

But remember, a decision to change physicians should be based on reality, and not on a quest to find a doctor who will tell you what you want to hear, or promise you a cure.

> **TOMMA**
>
> My son, who happens to be a doctor. The first thing he said is, "You need a second opinion. At a teaching medical center, with a whole team of doctors. Surgeons, oncologists, a nurse navigator."

TOMMA: You hear the "C" word, and the first thing you want to do is get rid of it. But it may be the wrong thing to do. Get the facts before you do anything. Check all your options.

GATHERING INFORMATION

The more you know, the more active you can be in your own care, and the more comfortable you will be with the decisions that are made. Becoming well informed about your treatment is one of the most important steps you can take at this time. A firm grasp of the facts will give you a sense of comfort and control.

Your main source of information will be the professionals caring for you. Make lists of topics you want to discuss, and don't hesitate to ask any question, no matter how simple it may seem. Ask your support person to accompany you to the medical appointments, so that you have someone to help you take notes, tape record what was said, or ask additional questions.

A lot of information—and, sadly, misinformation—is readily available on the internet. Be sure that the site you are consulting is managed by a reputable organization, and does not represent some individual's bias. If you

QUESTIONS TO ASK YOUR DOCTOR:

- **Is there a multidisciplinary lung cancer team in the facility where you practice?**

- **Could you give me the names of specialists you think I should see?**

- **How about another set of names so I can choose the specialist(s) I like best?**

- **Tell me about your, or your colleagues' experience in dealing with lung cancer.**

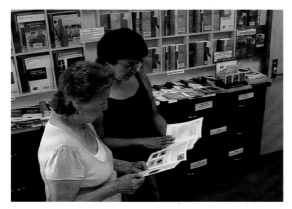

Ask your spouse, friend or partner to help you find the information you need.

have questions or concerns about any information you come across, let a member of your healthcare team know that you wish to discuss the information at your next appointment. Together you can evaluate what you read, and decide whether it is applicable to you.

On a regional or national level, there are organizations that can be valuable sources of information. Check the internet for the latest listings. The specialists at these organizations, many of whom are lung cancer survivors themselves, can answer many general questions about cancer, or send you written materials and information.

QUESTIONS TO ASK YOUR DOCTOR:

• **Could you forward my chart, test results, and my biopsy slides to the doctor who is going to give me a second opinion?**

• **Can you give me the name of a lung cancer expert who can give me a second opinion?**

As you delve deeper into your research, you will find that there is a whole network of both survivors and professionals who are committed to keeping track of the latest and the best in lung cancer treatments. Make every effort to hook into this network as soon as you can.

Despite all the benefits of information, there are many patients who are not comfortable knowing all the facts about their diagnosis. Knowing too much gives them anxiety and sleepless nights. If this is true for you, you may choose to ask your partner or support person to be the information gatherer, or even the decision maker. This is okay. Don't be critical of yourself if this approach meets your needs.

LINDA: You won't get all the answers from a single doctor. They all have different opinions, different skills. I have taken Ed to about twelve doctors so far. Knowledge gives me a sense of regaining some control over the situation.

PLANNING YOUR TREATMENT

Planning your treatment should involve the entire team of specialists who consulted on your case, as well as your spouse, partner or your loved ones.

As information about your case is collected, your team of healthcare professionals will review the information available, and discuss your case with you and among themselves. You'll probably meet with various team members several times, while they develop a recommendation for a course of treatment that's best suited to your case.

Many cancer centers schedule conferences called "Tumor Boards" where current cancer cases may be discussed by many different cancer specialists at the same time. Ask your healthcare team if they have a Tumor Board, and if your case can be presented. Take advantage of this. You will not only be getting a second opinion but a third, fourth or even fifth opinion.

The key thing to remember is that it is only you who is entitled to make the final decision. All the members of the team need to respect it. That's why it is so important for you to learn all you can about your disease. The more information you can gather before you begin treatment, the better you will feel about your decision, and the more active role you'll be able to take.

Don't worry if you feel confused by the new words and concepts that you will come across. Most people do find them confusing at first. Just keep asking questions.

In the upcoming days and weeks, as you explore this book, talk with your healthcare professionals, and gather more information, you will begin to acquire the knowledge you need to make informed decisions. Decisions that are right for you.

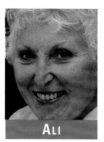

ALI

It was really depressing to gather information on the net, or even in books, because everything was so negative. It would have been nice to hear stories about people who survived ten, fifteen, twenty years. They are out there.

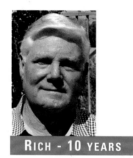

RICH - 10 YEARS

It is really important to choose one physician who will be the captain of your team. Who will know all about you, as a whole person. It may have saved me lots of complications down the line.

ED: When my doctor said, I have nothing available for you, I thought that meant no one had anything for me. Wrong! He meant in his puny little chemo infusion center. As soon as I started to look at other institutions, I found there were lots of options.

SPECIALISTS WHO MAY BE INVOLVED IN YOUR TREATMENT

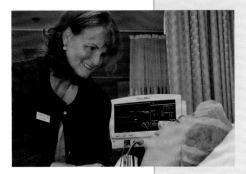

• **Anesthesiologist:** A physician who administers drugs or gasses which put you to sleep before surgery, and helps you with pain control after surgery.

• **Clinical Nurse Specialist:** A nurse with advanced training in a specific area, such as post-operative care, radiation or chemotherapy.

• **Medical Oncologist:** A physician who administers anti-cancer drugs or chemotherapy.

• **Nurse Navigator:** A specially trained nurse who will guide you through the maze of treatment options, helping you overcome obstacles with education and support.

• **Nutritionist:** A healthcare provider trained in nutrition and dietary counseling.

• **Oncology Social Worker:** A social worker who can provide counseling and practical assistance to cancer patience.

• **Pathologist:** A physician who examines the tissue removed during a biopsy, and issues a report to help you and your doctor choose the most effective treatment.

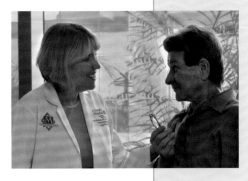

• **Personal Physician:** The doctor who will be responsible for coordinating your treatment. Your personal physician may be a surgeon, radiation oncologist, medical oncologist, or family physician.

• **Pulmonologist:** A physician who specializes in diagnosing and treating conditions affecting the respiratory system.

• **Physical Therapist:** A specialist who helps with post-surgical rehabilitation using exercise, heat, or massage.

• **Psychiatrist:** A physician who specializes in treating psychological conditions with psychotherapy and medications.

• **Psychologist:** A person trained in psychotherapy.

• **Radiation Oncologist:** A physician specially trained in using high energy X-rays for treatment.

• **Radiation Therapy Technologist:** A technologist who works under the direction of the Radiation Oncologist to administer radiation treatment.

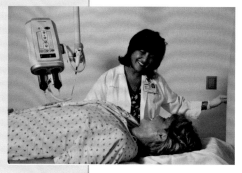

• **Respiratory Therapist:** A health professional who administers breathing treatments and helps your lungs perform as well as possible.

• **Social Worker:** A trained professional who can deal with social and economic aspects of treatment, such as helping find a support group or solving an insurance issue.

• **Surgeon:** A physician specializing in surgery, who will do the initial operation on the cancer. Many surgeons get additional training to become sub-specialists in chest surgery.

LEARN THE LINGO

Phrases commonly used to describe the result of therapy:

• **Complete response** – the tumor appears to be completely gone on the X-ray or scan, as a result of treatment.

• **Apparently cancer-free** – the tumor has disappeared after treatment.

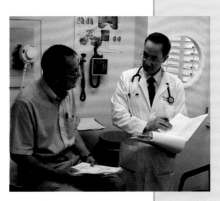

• **NED** – no evidence of disease.

• **Partial response** – the tumor has shrunk in size by at least 30%.

• **Stable disease** – the tumor did not grow or shrink noticeably.

• **Progressive disease** – the tumor is growing in spite of the treatment.

• **First-line therapy** – the first therapy used before any other treatments.

• **Second-line therapy** – treatment that may follow first-line therapy.

• **Multimodality or combined modality therapy** – the use of chemotherapy along with surgery, radiation therapy, targeted therapy or a combination.

• **Curative therapy** – is given with the intent or hope to completely cure the cancer.

• **Palliative therapy** – is given to relieve symptoms, provide better quality of life, and perhaps extend life when cure is not probable.

CHAPTER 2

LUNG CANCER BASICS

LUNG ANATOMY AND FUNCTION

Let's review the structure and function of the respiratory system. You know where the lungs are and what they do, but some of the terms like "lymph nodes" and "bronchi" may be new to you, and learning what they mean will help you understand lung cancer treatment better.

The main part of the respiratory system consists of two large, spongy structures—the *lungs*.

The right lung is made up of three parts, called *lobes*. The left lung is smaller to allow space for the heart. It is divided into two lobes.

Each lobe is subdivided into *segments*. One segment is equivalent to about one tenth of a lung. So when you have a segment resection as part of the treatment for lung cancer, your total lung capacity is decreased by about 5%. The partitions between segments make it easier to isolate the area of the lung where cancer is located.

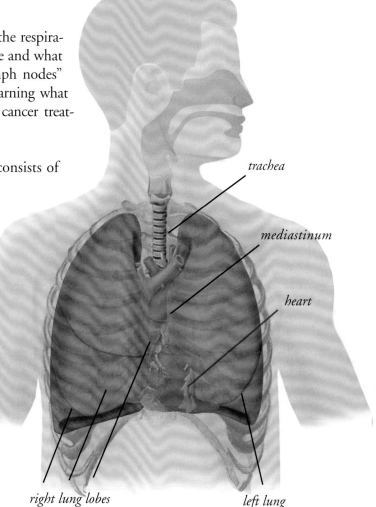

trachea

mediastinum

heart

right lung lobes

left lung

The space between the lungs is called the ***mediastinum***. It is located right under your sternum, or breast bone. In the mediastinum the trachea, bronchi, major arteries and lymph nodes are all crowded together, making surgery in this space very challenging.

Air enters the lungs through the nose and mouth, and travels down the windpipe, or ***trachea***.

right main stem bronchus

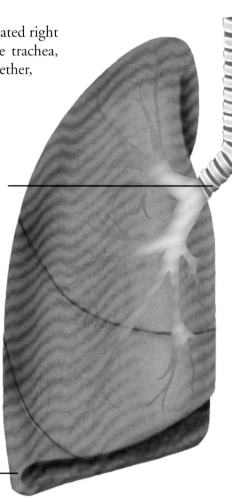

In the middle of the chest, the trachea branches into two smaller tubes, the right and left ***main stem bronchi***. (A reminder: "right" and "left" always refer to the point of view of the patient, facing forward. So the "right" lung will appear on the left side of a picture, or of an X-ray.)

Within the lungs the bronchi divide into smaller branches, the ***bronchioles***. The smallest bronchioles may be as thin as a hair.

The bronchioles end in millions of air sacs, called ***alveoli***.

lung section, magnified x30

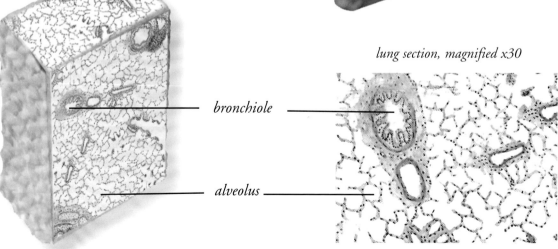

bronchiole

alveolus

A thin membrane called the *pleura* covers the outside of each lung and the inside of the chest. This creates a sac called the *pleural cavity.*

partially collapsed left lung

pleura, opened to show pleural cavity

The pleural cavity normally contains a small amount of fluid that helps the lungs move smoothly within the chest when you breathe.

The trachea and bronchi are kept semi-rigid and open by rings of cartilage. But the lungs themselves are soft, spongy organs that are kept inflated only by the vacuum that exists between the lungs and the rib cage and the diaphragm.

When there is a leakage of air or blood into the pleural cavity, the seal is broken, and one, or sometimes both, lungs collapse, leading to a respiratory emergency. You can better understand the concept if you think of a vacuum-packed bag of coffee. Pop the seal, and the whole package goes limp.

How does the oxygen-rich air get from the lungs to your organs? As air is inhaled, it reaches the alveoli, which are entertwined with a network of tiny blood vessels, the *capillaries.*

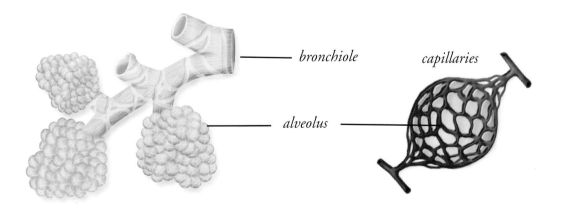

bronchiole

capillaries

alveolus

In the alveoli, the oxygen-rich blood releases oxygen molecules. The molecules are picked up by the red cells (the RBC's) in the blood, and carried to other parts of the body. At the same time, the blood unloads carbon dioxide molecules, that are then expelled into the air.

THE LYMPHATIC SYSTEM

lymph nodes

There is one more important component that will help you understand cancer treatment: the lymphatic system. *Lymph* is the fluid that naturally leaks out of the blood vessels and accumulates between cells. Lymph ducts collect this fluid and return it to the main circulation.

Along the way, lymphatic fluid is filtered through tiny bean-shaped structures called *lymph nodes*, which trap debris such as bacteria, or escaped cancer cells. You may think of the lymphatic system as a network of sewer lines with filter grids.

Most of the lymphatic fluid from the lungs drains toward the middle of the chest, the mediastinum, where it is filtered through the mediastinal lymph nodes. By examining the lymph nodes, the surgeon can get a good indication of whether cancer cells have begun to escape from the lungs toward the rest of the body. If the nodes are free of cancer cells, it is a good sign: the cancer has probably not spread beyond the lungs.

WHAT IS LUNG CANCER?

All organs in the body are made of *cells*. Individual cells are so small, they can only be seen through a microscope. Normal cells divide in an orderly fashion to replace cells that have aged and died. Controls within each cell tell it to stop dividing if no new cells are needed. The entire process is programmed into the genetic material within the cells, DNA.

Occasionally, damage to DNA during cell duplication may cause the controls to malfunction. Cells begin to divide uncontrollably, forming lumps or tumors.

Day one

Tumors

The word "*tumor*" comes from a Latin word that means "swelling." A tumor could be composed of cells that divide excessively, but that do not invade or damage other parts of the body. In this case the tumor is called a *benign*, that is, a non-cancerous, tumor.

On the other hand, a *malignant* tumor is composed of aggressively dividing cells that destroy surrounding tissues and travel to other parts of the body. In general conversation, the word "tumor" is often used to refer to a malignant condition, or cancer.

Growth Rate

Growth rate is the speed at which a tumor grows. Different types of cancer grow at different rates. The time it takes for a tumor to become twice as large is called doubling time. The average doubling time for most lung cancer tumors is in the range of 30 to 500 days, the average being 100 days.

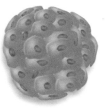

The change of the first normal cell into a malignant cell happens years before any evidence of cancer can be detected by a radiologic test such as a chest X-ray, chest CT scan or MRI. Lung cancer can stay so hidden that many people will not even know they have it until they experience symptoms such as coughing up blood, severe shortness of breath, or weight loss. In other words, by the time your cancer has been detected, it has been growing for several years.

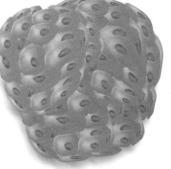

Two years later...

On average, the number of cells in a tumor doubles every 100 days

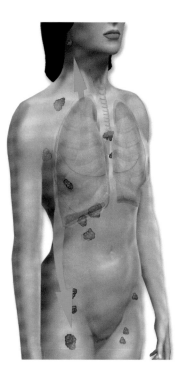

HOW CANCER SPREADS

As a malignant tumor grows, it may spread locally, invading and sometimes destroying adjacent tissues, or cells may break away from the tumor and get into the lymphatic vessels, or into the blood stream, and travel to distant parts of the body.

Some of the breakaway cells will be trapped in the lymph nodes in the mediastinum, or more distant areas. Examination of these nodes by a procedure called lymph node dissection, can help determine the stage (the degree of spread) of the cancer.

If cancer cells escape beyond the lymph nodes, or enter the circulatory system directly, they can spread to the liver, brain, and bones, forming new tumors called metastases. These distant metastases are the most worrisome, because they can damage vital organs. This advanced stage of cancer is called metastatic cancer, and its management is very difficult.

RISK FACTORS

Anything that increases a person's chance of developing a disease is called a *risk factor*. Having a risk factor does not mean that you will get cancer; not having risk factors doesn't mean that you won't.

Smoking cigarettes or cigars is the most common cause of lung cancer. The more years a person smokes, the greater the risk. If a person has stopped smoking, the risk becomes lower as the years pass, but is never completely gone.

RISK FACTORS FOR LUNG CANCER INCLUDE:

- Smoking cigarettes or cigars.
- Exposure to second-hand smoke.
- Past radiation therapy to the breast or chest area.
- Exposure to asbestos, radon, chromium, arsenic, soot, or tar.
- Environmental factors such as air pollution.
- Family history of lung cancer.

s lung cancer hereditary? Researchers found that people who have a first-degree relative with lung cancer have nearly double the risk of developing lung cancer themselves. This is a factor to bear in mind when you tell your relatives about your diagnosis. They may consider being more vigilant in the future.

TYPES OF LUNG CANCER

Lung cancers are divided into two major types: *non-small cell lung cancer* (NSCLC) and *small cell lung cancer* (SCLC). These names may be confusing to a layman, but they refer to the appearance of the cells under the microscope. NSCLC cells are bigger than SCLC cells.

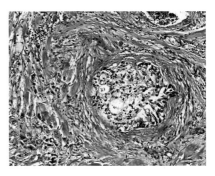

Non-small cell lung cancers account for about eight of ten cases of lung cancer. Non-small cell lung cancers can be of several types, and are similar to one another in how they grow, spread, or respond to treatment. That is why they are grouped together as NSCLCs.

Adenocarcinoma is now the most common form of non-small cell lung cancer. It is found in smokers and non-smokers. It starts in the inside border of the lungs and can be present for a long time before it is detected.

Squamous cell carcinoma used to be more common, but now accounts for roughly 30% of non-small cell lung cancers in the United States. It usually starts in the bronchial tubes, in the middle of the lungs, and commonly is found after individuals begin to cough up blood. Some experts feel that filtered cigarettes have caused the decline in squamous cell lung cancer and that adenocarcinoma is more common now since toxins are inhaled deeper into the lungs.

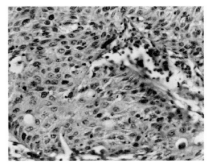

Large cell cancers are less common accounting for up to 10% of non-small cell lung cancers in the United States. They occur in the outer edges of the lungs and tend to grow rapidly.

The third type, large cell carcinoma, is actually a form of adenocarcinoma, but the cells look much larger under a microscope. This type of lung cancer occurs in the outer edges of the lungs and tends to grow rapidly.

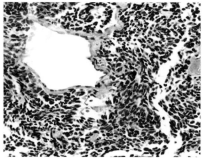

Small cell lung cancer used to be called "oat cell carcinoma". About two out of every ten lung cancers diagnosed are of this type. This type of cancer is almost always caused by smoking. It is very rare for someone who has never smoked to develop it.

Small cell carcinoma is different from non-small cell carcinoma in that it often spreads quite early. Because of this, it is usually diagnosed at a more advanced stage, when it has already spread throughout the lungs or body. It is however, very sensitive to chemotherapy.

Your physician will tell you whether you have SCLC (small cell lung cancer) or NSCLC (non-small cell lung cancer). Remember which type of cancer you have as you go through the book so you can concentrate on the information most relevant to your case.

●●●

Now you know most of the anatomy words and concepts you will need to understand your treatment. Soon they will become part of your daily vocabulary.

CHAPTER 3

DIAGNOSIS AND STAGING

DIAGNOSIS

Chances are that if you are reading this book, you've already had a biopsy that showed that your tumor is lung cancer. If so, feel free to skip to the Staging section of this chapter.

Lung cancer is not easy to find early. Usually the physician will suspect it if the patient, especially a smoker, has a persistent or worsening cough, shortness of breath, bloody sputum, or other respiratory changes. Occasionally, the first clue of something abnormal is a small shadow detected on a chest X-ray or scan done for other reasons, such as before surgery.

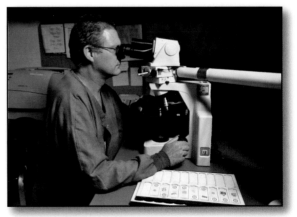

The first test in attempting to pinpoint the problem will be a chest X-ray, but often the tumor is so small that it does not register on a conventional chest X-ray.

A pathologist identifies the tissue under a microscope

Next, a CT scan may be recommended since CT scans can detect tumors too small to be seen on X-rays, and reveal whether the lymph nodes inside the chest are enlarged – a warning sign that cancer may have begun to spread.

Magnetic resonance imaging (MRI), or techniques such as PET-CT scanners which combine the PET and CT technology in one machine, may yield even more valuable information.

Biopsy

The only way to confirm the diagnosis of cancer is with a *biopsy*—taking a sample of tissue directly from the suspected lesion and sending it to a pathologist for examination under the microscope.

One way to obtain a sample of lung tissue is with *bronchoscopy*. A tube with a light and camera at the tip is inserted into the bronchi through the airway, and advanced all the way to the lesion. A sampling device at the end of the bronchoscope snips and retrieves a small piece of tissue.

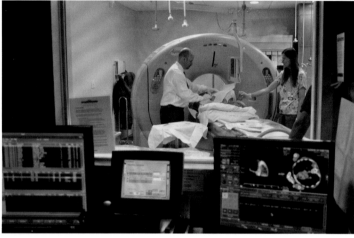

Biopsy with CT guidance

Courtesy Pomona Valley Hospital

Another technique is *needle biopsy*. A surgeon inserts a needle through the skin and using CT for guidance, obtains a sample of the tissue. This biopsy is performed with a device that works like an ear-piercing instrument: it propels a large needle very rapidly through the lesion. A special notch in the needle traps a sliver of tissue for examination. Samples obtained with core biopsy are large enough to be cut into thin slices for detailed examination under the microscope.

Endobronchial ultrasound, or EBUS, is a minimally invasive procedure similar to a bronchoscopy, but assisted by an ultrasound device. It is a good alternative for patients who cannot tolerate a surgical biopsy.

Instead of a cell sample, a *liquid biopsy* can sometimes be used. It is based on evaluation of a blood sample, which is more easily obtainable than a tissue biopsy.

One of the most important pieces of information about your disease is the type of lung cancer that you have. This identification is made by the pathologist based on what the cells of the tumor look like. The results will be communicated to your surgeon within days, and will indicate whether you have NSCLC or SCLC.

GENOMIC TESTING

Each person's cancer has a unique combination of genetic changes. Analyzing the tumor to identify these changes is called DNA sequencing, or genetic or genomic testing. Tests developed in the past few years can be very valuable in deciding whether a particular tumor will respond to a specific treatment.

The results can help your healthcare team predict your chances that the cancer might come back, and identify the most effective therapies for successful treatment. Ask your health care provider to discuss the possibility of tumor DNA sequencing, also knows as *genomic testing* or molecular analysis, as part of your care.

Sometimes treatment can cause a tumor makeup to change or the tumor to become resistant to targeted therapy. Ask your doctor about re-testing your tumor after your first treatment.

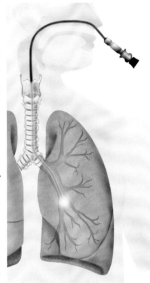

Bronchoscope inserted through the trachea

Personalized Medicine

Cancer specialists are now using these gene-based diagnostic tests in various ways to plan more effective treatments. Tests that analyze dozens of genes in the tumor help doctors create treatment plans that are personalized to your particular case. This approach is also called precision medicine.

Genomic testing is rapidly becoming the foundation and the gold standard of "personalized medicine".

STAGING

Why Staging?

Each cancer is unique, each patient is different, and the combination of treatment options is practically endless. To help determine who should get what treatment, cancer specialists rely on staging—a system that places the cancer into a certain group. The stage of your tumor is the most important factor in deciding what type of treatment is best for you.

A biopsy can confirm that the diagnosis is cancer, but it will not show whether the cancer has spread to other parts of the body. Additional tests and procedures may include the following:

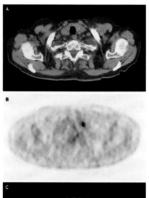

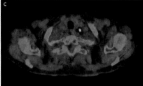

MRI

MRI or Magnetic Resonance Imaging uses a combination of magnetic energy and ordinary radio waves to create detailed images of the inside of your body.

Because the MRI unit can feel cramped, notify the technologist or your physician if you feel uncomfortable in confined spaces. MRI is painless, and does not expose you to X-ray radiation. The test takes about an hour.

CT Scan

CAT scan, CT scan, or Computerized Axial Tomography all mean the same thing. This test uses ordinary X-rays, and a rotating system to obtain detailed images of your body. The test is short and painless.

PET Scan

Lung cancer cells may metastasize, or spread, to distant organs. The most effective way to find these metastases is to perform a PET scan, which stands for Positron Emission Tomography scan.

For this scan, tiny amounts of radioactive substance are injected into a vein. The radioactive substance concentrates in areas where there is an unusually increased number of blood vessels—a "hot spot"—that may correspond to a new growth of cancer cells. A special camera creates an image that pinpoints the location of these hot spots.

PET/CT Scan

A PET/CT scan combines the ability of a PET scan to identify rapidly growing clusters of cells, with the CT's ability to image fine detail.

By combining the two images, a PET/CT scan will help determine whether the lung cancer has spread, especially to the liver, adrenal glands, or brain.

Mediastinoscopy

Mediastinoscopy is a procedure used to examine the tissues and lymph nodes in the mediastinum--the space that lies between the lungs. Under general anesthesia, the surgeon will make a small incision at the top of the breastbone and insert a tube-like instrument equipped with a light, a video lens, and a biopsy device.

Sampling the tissues and lymph nodes will enable your medical team to decide whether surgery should be recommended.

The Pathology Report

Clinical staging is the initial and tentative staging that is based on the results of the physical exam and the diagnostic tests performed before surgery.

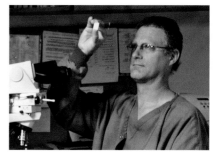

The final determination of the stage, called pathological staging, will come after the surgeon has an opportunity to examine the inside of the chest during the procedure, and the tumor and lymph nodes have been removed and examined under a microscope.

The final pathology report will specify the size of the tumor, the type of cell the tumor is composed of, and whether there is tumor spread to lymph nodes. This information is essential for planning your treatment.

Some patients consider the waiting for the final version of the pathologist's report to be one of the most stressful aspects of the cancer experience. There is nothing worse than being in limbo, but try to be patient. Remember that you will feel better once you have the final diagnosis and are able to start your treatment.

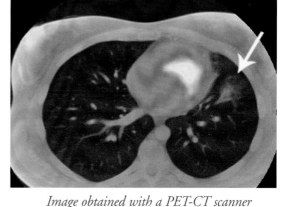

Image obtained with a PET-CT scanner
Courtesy Johnson Lightfoote, MD

STAGES OF NSCLC AND SCLC

Small cell and non-small cell cancers are staged differently because they behave differently. Remember what type of cancer you have so you can concentrate your attention on the information that is more relevant in your case.

Let's look at NSCLC stages first.

QUESTIONS TO ASK
YOUR DOCTOR:

- **What type of cancer do I have?**

- **What is the size of the tumor?**

- **What kind of tests will help determine if the cancer has spread?**

NON-SMALL CELL LUNG CANCER STAGING

TNM is the most common staging system for NSCLC. In simplified form, staging for this class of cancer is based on: the size of the tumor; presence of cancer cells in the lymph nodes; and metastasis, or spread, to other organs. This is the so-called TNM—tumor, node, metastasis—staging system.

Tumor size is determined when the tumor is removed and sent to the pathologist. The size is designated "is" (in situ) through 4. For example, a T2 tumor is 3 cm or larger—a bit bigger than an inch.

Lymph nodes are checked for evidence of tumor spread with preoperative scans, or at the time of surgery in a procedure called lymph node dissection. Lymph node spread is labeled 0-3. So N0 means no lymph node involvement.

Metastasis, or spread to other organs, is assessed with bone scans, CT scans, and PET-CT studies. Putting all this information together is called staging. M can be 0 or 1a or 1b. M0 means no metastases.

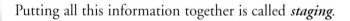

Putting all this information together is called *staging*.

Stages for NSCLC range from Stage 0, or occult, to Stage IV. (Beyond Stage 0 and Stage "is", stages are identified either by Roman numerals, I-IV or by Arabic numerals, 1-4). Each stage is further divided according to various factors (e.g. IIB or 3A, etc).

A Stage 0 tumor is described as TisN0M0. It is still confined (in situ) and has no known spread to lymph nodes (N0) or metastases (M0) to other parts of the body.

A Stage IIIB tumor can be either T4N2M0 or T1a-4N3M0. In other words, the tumor is bigger than 7 cm (almost 3 inches), is surrounded by satellite nodules, and has spread to lymph nodes, but not yet to distant parts of the body. And so on.

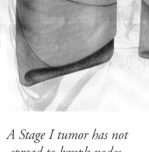

A Stage I tumor has not spread to lymph nodes.

If you are getting the impression that the actual determination of stage can be rather complex, you are right.

Needless to say, you don't need to figure out your own staging to understand your treatment options. Ask your physician to show you how she determined the stage of your cancer. With this information in hand, you will be able to participate actively in the treatment decision process.

As a quick overview, you may find it helpful to think of stage as degree of risk presented by a particular tumor:

At one end of the scale are the low-risk situations: very tiny tumors that have not spread to lymph nodes, and that are composed of cells that are not very aggressive.

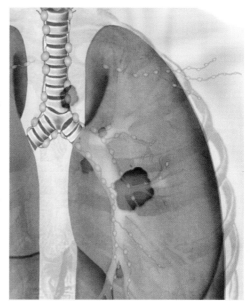

A Stage III tumor invaded a bronchus and spread to lymph nodes.

Further along are larger tumors, slightly bigger than an inch in size, (3 cm), that have spread to the main bronchus or the lung lining.

At the other end of the scale are the situations that involve the greatest risk: tumors that have invaded the lymph nodes, or spread to other organs.

If you are at the low-risk end of the scale, your treatment may require surgical removal of the tumor, perhaps followed by chemotherapy. Larger tumors may be treated with more aggressive chemotherapy. For high-risk tumors, at the far end of the scale, there are a wide variety of options, including radiation and chemotherapy.

All of these options are discussed in the Treatment Options chapter.

You may use special staging tables to determine your stage, but odds are that you will find that the task is quite complex because of the many different variables that must be taken into consideration.

A better option is to ask your healthcare team to guide you through the process.

NON-SMALL CELL LUNG CANCER STAGING

Stage 1

- Stage 1A: The cancer is smaller than 3cm, has not spread to the lymph nodes.
- Stage 1B: The cancer is larger than 3cm, or growing into a main bronchus. The cancer may also have spread to the pleura.

Stage 2

- Stage 2A: The cancer measures 3cm or less, and affects nearby lymph nodes.
- Stage 2B: The cancer is larger than 3cm and in the nearby lymph nodes, or no cancer in lymph nodes, but the tumor has made the lung collapse; or tumor has grown into chest wall, pleura, diaphragm, or pericardium.

Stage 3

- Stage 3A: Any size and spread into the lymph nodes in the mediastinum, but not to the other side of the chest or has spread to nearby tissue such as chest wall, pleura, mediastinum, etc.

- Stage 3B: The cancer has spread to lymph nodes on either side of the chest or above either collar bone there are two or more tumors in the same lung.

- Stage 4: The cancer has spread to a distant part of the body, such as the liver, bones, adrenal glands, or the brain.

SMALL CELL LUNG CANCER STAGING

In contrast to NSCLC staging, SCLC staging is about as simple as it gets. There are only two stages: limited and extensive.

The reason the staging is different for the two types is that at diagnosis the small cell cancers are generally at an advanced stage, and so the I-IV classification would not be useful.

SMALL CELL LUNG CANCER STAGING

Limited Stage: The cancer is found in one lung, in the tissues between the lungs, and in nearby lymph nodes only.

Extensive Stage: The cancer has spread from the lung in which it began into the other lung, or to other parts of the body.

•••

I don't mean to belabor the point, but I do want you to understand how important correct staging is for your treatment.

Medical researchers are constantly evaluating the benefits of various treatments. What works in Stage 3A, might not work for a 3B tumor. What was standard therapy for Stage 2A last year, might have been replaced with better options today.

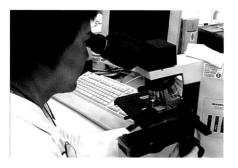

By accurately determining the stage of your cancer, your medical team can make the best recommendations, based on the latest information—and improve your chances of successful treatment.

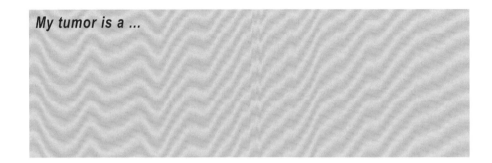

My tumor is a ...

The stage of MY tumor is ...

CHAPTER 4

TREATMENT OPTIONS

UNDERSTANDING TREATMENT OPTIONS

The treatment options available to you depend on the type, location and stage of your lung cancer, as well as on your age, general health, pre-existing diseases or conditions, and your ability to tolerate the side effects of treatment.

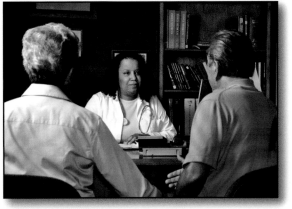

It is important to know if you have been diagnosed with non-small cell lung cancer (NSCLC) or small cell lung cancer (SCLC), because your treatment options will be different.

Surgery, radiation therapy, chemotherapy and targeted therapy are the primary tools for treating lung cancer. Depending on the extent of the cancer, these therapies can be used alone or in combination with each other to achieve more effective results.

After a simplified overview of the various treatment types, we will look at the specific options available for patients with SCLC and NSCLC, stage by stage. The options are not the same, because the two types of cancer are usually detected at different stages. The various therapies will be described in greater detail in the following chapters.

After you find out what type of lung cancer you have, and review the general information, feel free to skip to the section that applies to your specific cancer.

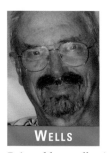

WELLS

Being able to talk with your doctors is key. If you can't, get yourself a support partner who can. Talk about the treatments. Question everything. Evaluate results. Change course if necessary.

SURGERY

Surgery is the oldest and still the most common way to manage most types of lung cancer. The goal is to remove the entire tumor, plus enough tissue that appears free of cancer around it to be reasonably sure that no cancer cells are left behind.

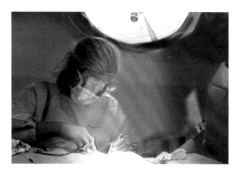

The various surgical procedures are named according to how much of the lung is removed. A *wedge resection* removes the tumor and some of the normal tissue around it. A *lobectomy* removes the whole lobe, while a *bilobectomy* removes two lobes. A *pneumonectomy* removes the entire lung. We will describe each in more detail in the Surgery Chapter.

Surgery is more effective in early-stage non–small cell lung cancer when the tumor has not spread to lymph nodes or outside the chest cavity, and it is small enough to be removed.

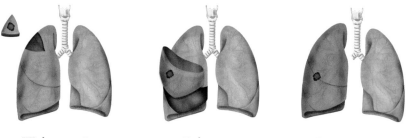

Wedge resection   *Lobectomy*   *Pneumonectomy*

Surgery is used in a small minority of limited-stage small cell lung cancer if the cancer happened to be diagnosed at a very early stage, when it was still very small.

Surgery would not be useful for advanced cancer that has spread to various areas of both lungs.

RADIATION THERAPY

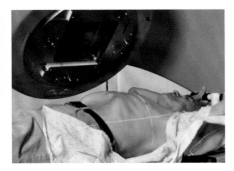

Radiation therapy uses high-energy X-rays to kill cancer cells. The goal is to deliver the most effective dose of radiation to the tumor, while limiting the damage to surrounding normal tissues. The way the radiation therapy is given depends on the type and stage of the cancer being treated.

QUESTIONS TO ASK
YOUR DOCTOR:

- **What is the goal of my treatment – attempt to cure, or manage symptoms and improve quality of life?**

- **Do you have a team of doctors working with you on my case? If not, why not?**

There are two ways to administer radiation therapy.

External beam radiation therapy uses a machine outside the body to send radiation toward the cancer. The machine aims the radiation beams from different angles in order to cut down on the damage to normal tissues in the area. Treatments are generally given daily for several weeks, with rest days on weekends.

Lung cancers pose a challenge to radiation therapy because the rise and fall of the abdomen and lungs during breathing makes the tumors difficult to target. *Stereotactic Radiosurgery* is a method of delivering very high doses of radiation to the tumor, directly and precisely, with little damage to healthy tissue. The method relies on implanting tiny metal "seeds" in the tumor, enabling the machinery to follow movement and deliver radiation when the tumor is in the precise position necessary. Treatment courses are generally completed in one-to-five days.

Internal radiation therapy, also called *brachytherapy*, uses radioactive substances sealed in needles, seeds or catheters that are placed directly into or near the cancer. Brachytherapy treatments can be given over a few days. The shorter time commitments are appreciated by patients who live far from the hospital.

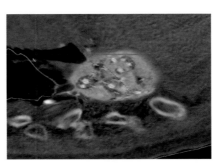

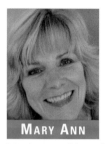

MARY ANN

My doctor told me, "Don't think about your symptoms, except when you come to see me. That's it. Live normally." That was probably the best advice I ever got!

CHEMOTHERAPY

Chemotherapy uses drugs, called *cytotoxic* (cell-killing) drugs, to stop the growth of cancer cells, or to destroy them.

The drugs are injected into the blood stream, and travel to reach cancer cells almost anywhere in the body. The way the chemotherapy is given depends on the type and stage of the cancer being treated.

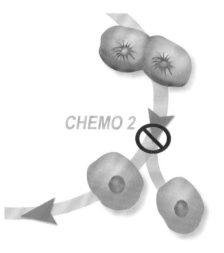

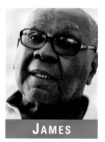

JAMES

They just started using targeted therapy when I was diagnosed - so I got the benefit of a brand new treatment.

TARGETED THERAPY

Targeted therapy is a promising approach to cancer treatment that is designed to target cancer cells specifically.

Substances made by the body or made in a laboratory are used to boost, direct, or restore the body's natural defenses against cancer.

Targeted therapy works differently from cell-killing chemotherapy and has different and less severe side effects.

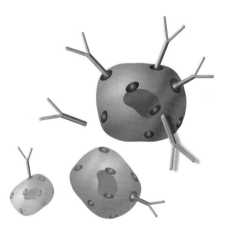

IMMUNOTHERAPY

Immunotherapy is perhaps the most promising recent development in lung cancer treatment. The approach relies on substances that manipulate the patient's own immune system to aggressively attack cancer cells.

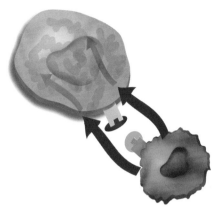

Because the side effects of immune-boosting drugs are relatively benign compared with those of chemotherapy, it's possible for some patients to stay on them for many years to keep their lung cancer under control

OTHER THERAPIES

There is a number of approaches that can be used to either attempt to cure the cancer, or to relieve the symptoms.

Photodynamic therapy (PDT) or Laser Therapy

Photodynamic therapy (PDT) uses a combination of a drug plus a type of laser. A drug that is not active until it is exposed to light is injected into a vein. The drug collects more in cancer cells than in normal cells, which have a much slower growth cycle. Fiberoptic tubes are then used to carry the laser light to the cancer area, where the drug becomes active and kills the cells.

Radiofrequency Ablation (RFA)

RFA can be used to treat patients whose health excludes the possibility of surgery, or who have tumors that are inoperable. The procedure is done as an outpatient, under conscious sedation (light sleep). Electrodes are used to heat and destroy the tumor.

Clinical Trials

Scientists are constantly searching for better ways of dealing with cancer. This search is done in the form of clinical trials. A clinical trial is an evaluation of a new way of managing cancer—with a new drug, a new procedure or a new diagnostic tool.

For some patients, taking part in a clinical trial may be the best treatment choice. Clinical trials are taking place in many parts of the country. Ask your medical team to discuss the clinical trials options available to you.

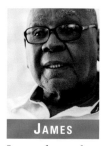

JAMES

I wanted to evaluate all the aspects of the treatments they were proposing. So I took my time. It drove my family nuts, because they wanted me to get on with it.

TREATMENT OPTIONS BY STAGE

To get a bird's eye view, you may think of treatment choices this way:

Non-small cell lung cancer—NSCLC—may be treated with surgery plus radiation therapy, with chemotherapy and with targeted therapy.

Small cell lung cancer—SCLC—is usually treated with radiation therapy and chemotherapy.

Now let's see how the treatments apply by stage. You may notice that the more advanced the cancer stage, the more varied the options.

NSCLC	SCLC
Surgery	*Radiation Therapy*
Radiation Therapy	*Chemotherapy*
Chemotherapy	
Targeted Therapy	

ED: So many patients are very ill informed. They are happy to do what the first doctor says. Ask them, "What kind of lung cancer do you have?"   "I don't know."   "What stage are you?" "I don't know." "Who won American Idol?" That they know. It's a shame. Your job number one should be to stay informed!

I don't care if you are educated, a scientist, or a blue collar worker. You have to become an expert in your disease. Your doctors need your help!! They will help you if you help them.

Non-Small Cell Lung Cancer

Occult
Can usually be cured by surgery, depending on the location.

Stage 0 (carcinoma in situ)
Surgery (wedge resection or segmental resection) or
Photodynamic therapy using an endoscope.

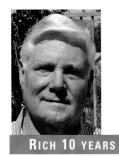

RICH 10 YEARS

They were planning on minimally invasive, but after I was asleep they decided I needed a whole lobe resected. So now I can't ride my bike 100 miles anymore. Miss that piece of lung.

Stage I
Surgery (wedge resection, segmental resection, or lobectomy).
External radiation therapy for patients who can't have surgery.
Surgery followed by chemotherapy.
A clinical trial of photodynamic therapy using an endoscope.
A clinical trial of surgery followed by chemoprevention.

Stage II
Surgery (wedge or segmental resection, lobectomy or pneumonectomy).
External radiation therapy for patients who can't have surgery.
Surgery followed by chemotherapy with or without other treatments.
A clinical trial of external radiation therapy following surgery.

Stage III
Surgery with or without radiation therapy.
External radiation therapy alone.
Chemotherapy combined with other treatments.
A clinical trial of radiation therapy and chemotherapy.
Chemotherapy combined with external radiation therapy.

Stage IV
A clinical trial of chemotherapy with or without biologic therapy.
Chemotherapy.
External radiation therapy to relieve pain and improve the quality of life.
Laser therapy and/or internal radiation therapy.

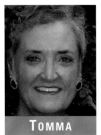

TOMMA

Good thing I waited. If I had started on something, it would have excluded me from being able to participate in the clinical trial that I entered later.

Small Cell Lung Cancer

Limited-Stage

Chemotherapy and radiation therapy.

Chemotherapy alone for patients who are very ill.

Surgery only occasionally, since SCLC is seldom diagnosed at an early stage.

Surgery, then chemotherapy, or chemotherapy plus radiation therapy.

Clinical trials of new chemotherapy, surgery, and radiation treatments.

Extensive-Stage

Combination chemotherapy.

Radiation therapy to the brain may later be given.

Radiation therapy to the brain, or other parts of the body as palliative therapy to relieve symptoms and improve quality of life.

Clinical trials of new chemotherapy treatments.

●●●

PERSONALIZED MEDICINE

Cancer specialists are now using gene-based diagnostic tests in various ways to plan more effective treatments for patients with lung cancer. These tests analyze dozens of genes in the tumor to help patients and their doctors make decisions about whether or not to include chemotherapy in their treatment plan.

WELLS: People say that survival statistics haven't changed. That might be true, but in my ten years plus in lung cancer, I have seen a tremendous change in how treatment is approached. It is more personalized. We are relying more on genetic testing to make treatment more tailored. Things have changed. Soon we will have genetic profiling like we have in breast cancer for example.

CHAPTER 5

SURGERY

SURGERY

To ensure the best chance of successful treatment of lung cancer, it is important to remove the entire tumor, using the most direct approach possible.

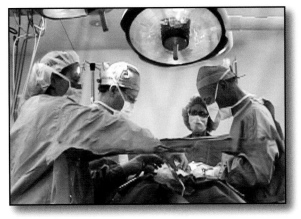

Surgery is the gold standard for early stage non-small cell lung cancer (NSCLC). Usually, a small, localized, NSCLC tumor can be surgically removed, with an excellent outlook for a cure.

Surgery can sometimes be used for larger, later stage NSCLC tumors after they are shrunk by chemotherapy or by radiation therapy.

Surgery on late stage NSCLC is not always an option, and will have to be determined by your medical team.

Surgery is not usually used to treat SCLC (small cell lung cancer) because by the time this type of cancer is diagnosed, it usually has spread to more than one place in the body. Surgery can sometimes be used in very early stage SCLC, when the tumor is tiny.

Other treatments, such as radiation therapy or chemotherapy, may play an important role in the treatment plan, either in conjunction with, or instead of, surgery. These methods will be discussed in other chapters.

QUESTIONS TO ASK
YOUR SURGEON:

- What type of procedure do you think is best for me?

- What is the latest information about this type of cancer surgery?

- Could I meet with some of the patients who had this procedure before?

SURGICAL PROCEDURES

Surgical procedures for lung cancer are named according to the amount of lung removed.

Lobectomy

A lobectomy is the "standard of care" for patients with lung cancer who can be treated with surgery. In other words, most reputable surgeons consider lobectomy to be the treatment of choice, if the patient is strong enough to tolerate surgery.

The procedure involves removal of a lobe of the lung. At the same time, the surgeon will examine the lymph nodes in the mediastinum for evidence of cancer spread.

A bilobectomy removes two lobes. It can be done only on the right lung which has three lobes.

Pneumonectomy

A pneumonectomy removes the entire lung. Your specialist will recommend this operation if the position of the tumor is central within the lung and involves either both lobes on the left or the three lobes on the right. Your pre-operative pulmonary function tests will determine how well you will be able to function with one of your lungs removed. Most patients can lead a normal life with only one lung if it is a healthy one.

The surgical approach usually involves making an incision across the side of the chest and spreading the ribs to gain access to the lung. This is called a thoracotomy.

Wedge Resections and Segmentectomies

Wedge resections and segmentectomies ("segment removal") are used less commonly in the surgical treatment of lung cancer. These procedures are done only on tiny cancers, and only in patients who cannot undergo a full lobectomy.

The advantage of a lobectomy is that it removes a generous portion of lung tissue around the tumor. This decreases the chances that any cancerous cells are left behind. Unfortunately, it also decreases your breathing reserves. If your lungs are weak before surgery, you might not be able to afford losing any more breathing capacity.

By performing a wedge resection or a segmentectomy, the surgeon can save more lung tissue. And that might give you enough of a breathing advantage, so that you can be treated with surgery, rather than settling for a less effective treatment.

VATS

Usually, wedge resections and lobectomies are performed by removing the diseased part of the lung through small incisions, with the help of a video camera. This is called Video-Assisted Thoracic Surgery, or VATS.

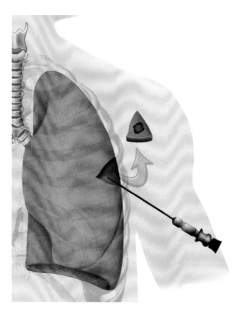

Video-Assisted Lung Cancer Surgery (or minimally invasive lung cancer surgery) offers several benefits, including a shorter hospital stay, less pain and earlier return to usual activities. It is now the "standard of care" for early lung cancers.

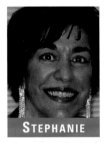

STEPHANIE

Honestly, I think they didn't quite warn me. Having my lung taken out was ten times more painful than giving birth.

QUESTIONS TO ASK
YOUR SURGEON:

• How much pain should I expect after the procedure?

• How long before I can go back to my regular work or leisure activities?

• Will there be any long term effects?

• What follow-up visits do you recommend?

• How long can I take narcotics for pain without getting addicted?

Getting Ready

Depending on the extent of your cancer, you may require the removal of just a small piece of the lung, a lobe of the lung, or the entire lung. No matter how seemingly simple the operation, it will involve general anesthesia, an incision across your breathing muscles, post-operative pain, and other significant disruption to your breathing.

To make sure that your general health is up to the challenge, your medical team will recommend a number of tests.

These tests will include blood tests to make sure you are not anemic, and that your liver and kidneys are functioning properly. You will have an ECG (electrocardiogram) to check for past or present heart damage.

PRE-OP CHECKLIST

• Stop smoking, and using recreational drugs and alcohol

• Stop all medications that interfere with blood clotting, such as aspirin, Advil, Motrin, etc.

• Ask your internist about stoppage of blood thinners

• Stop taking vitamins, unless approved by the surgeon

• Check your health and disability benefits

• Recruit help and schedule time off

You will also have breathing tests, called *pulmonary function tests* or *spirometry*. These tests will measure how much air you can breathe in and out, and how much reserve you have to get you through the post-surgical recovery.

Sometime before your surgery, a respiratory therapist will teach you how to perform *breathing exercises* that will help you avoid lung infections, and recover more quickly. You will also learn leg exercises to prevent blood clots from forming while you are lying in bed, recuperating.

Pre-Operative Details

After the surgery date is set, someone on your surgeon's staff will review with you the admission process for the particular hospital where the operation will take place. Find out whether your insurance covers surgical fees, hospital room, anesthesiologist's fees, and other charges.

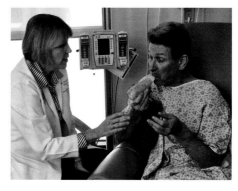

Make a list of all the medications you are taking, both prescription and over-the-counter, since some of them may have adverse effects during anesthesia or surgery. (For example, aspirin-containing preparations can increase bleeding.) Some medications may need to be discontinued several weeks before surgery. Be sure to mention your allergies, colds, and oral issues, such as dentures or tooth decay.

If you haven't stopped smoking, do so, even if just to give your lungs a fighting chance for recovering after surgery. Ideally, you should stop smoking six weeks before your lung surgery.

STOP SMOKING BEFORE SURGERY

Ask your healthcare provider for help in quitting smoking. She may be able to prescribe nicotine replacement therapy (NRT), or recommend one of the many over-the-counter products available. These products, combined with behavioral modifications, will double your chance of quitting smoking—and greatly increase your ability to tolerate lung surgery.

Blood transfusions are rarely required during lung surgery. You may wish to discuss with your physician the possibility of donating and storing your own blood before your surgery so that it can be used should you need it. You will need to donate the blood at least one week before surgery.

QUESTIONS TO ASK YOUR ANESTHESIOLOGIST:

- **Will you give me something to help me relax before the procedure?**
- **How long will it take me to get back to normal after the sedation?**
- **What are the side effects of sedation?**
- **If I have general anesthesia, how long will it take me to get back to normal?**
- **Will you give me something to control the pain after I wake up from the anesthetic?**

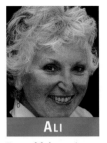

ALI

I wouldn't say it was terrible.
To compare to my three
C-sections, I would say it
was worse, probably because
they cut a lot of the breathing muscles.

Pack all the personal belongings you may need: a nightgown or pajamas, slippers, toiletries, books or an iPod, perhaps a favorite pillow, and a change of loose, easy to don, clothing to wear when you go home.

Most people undergoing surgery enjoy having a friend or relative accompany them to the hospital and meet them after the procedure. When you are discharged to go home, you will definitely need someone to drive you.

Surgery Day

You'll be instructed not to eat or drink anything after midnight on the night before the surgery.

On the day of the surgery, you'll first go through an admission process at the hospital. The hospital staff will ask you to sign an informed consent form listing your doctor's name and the name of the surgical procedure you are having. Make sure you feel comfortable with what you are signing. If there is anything on the form that worries you, ask to see your doctor. Your surgeon will probably greet you in the pre-op area and reassure you about the outcome.

The pre-operative nurse will start an intravenous line (an "IV") in one of your arms using a small needle, and perhaps give you something to help you relax. The anesthesiologist will give you general anesthesia through your IV during surgery.

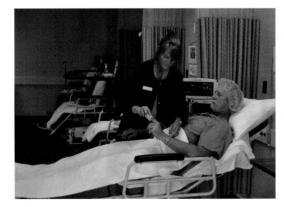

The anesthesiologist or the nurse anesthetist will talk to you prior to surgery and let you know your options for pain control after surgery when general anesthesia wears off. You may be offered an epidural (spinal block) to help with pain control following surgery. Or you may be offered patient-controlled analgesia (PCA)—a device that will deliver pain medication when you push a button.

The Surgical Procedure

When the surgical team is ready, you will be taken to the operating room. Several devices will be attached to your body, such as an automatic blood pressure cuff, a heart monitor, and a blood oxygen monitor.

The anesthesiologist will inject a drug into your vein through the tubing, and you will fall asleep almost immediately.

At that time, a tube will be placed through your mouth into the trachea to maintain a way for you to breathe during the surgery.

Your blood pressure, pulse, and breathing will be closely monitored during the entire procedure.

Depending on the procedure, the operation can take from one hour to three or four hours. The approach to the cancer, and the amount of lung tissue removed, will depend on the size of your tumor, on the suspected spread of the tumor, and on the position of the tumor relative to critical organs such as the heart and windpipe.

Depending on what the surgeon finds as the procedure progresses, the approach may change. For example, if the original plan was to perform a lobectomy (removing one lobe), but the surgeon finds that the cancer spread further than expected, a bilobectomy, (removal of two lobes) or even a pneumonectomy (removal of the entire lung) may be required.

The tissue removed will be sent to the pathologist, who will examine it for any evidence of cancer spread beyond the portion removed. If no cancer cells are found along the edges of the specimen, it will be described as having "clear margins", and the surgeon will be able to assume that the cancer has not spread into the adjacent lung tissue.

If cancer cells are found in the margins of the specimen, (the margins are "positive"), odds are that the tumor has spread beyond what was removed, and the surgeon will make a decision whether to remove more tissue, or resort to non-surgical therapy, such as radiation or chemotherapy.

QUESTIONS TO ASK YOUR SURGEON:

- **Do I need to arrange to have someone to help me with daily activities?**

- **How long before I can go back to my regular work or leisure activities?**

QUESTIONS TO ASK YOUR SURGEON:

- **How much lung will be removed?**

- **How will the removal of lung tissue affect my breathing?**

- **How much pain should I expect in the first few days after the procedure?**

Lymph Node Examination

Prior to your lung surgery, you may also undergo a procedure called a *mediastinoscopy*, to check for cancer spread beyond the lung to lymph nodes in the center of your chest, the mediastinum.

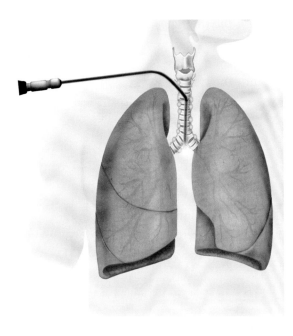

Why examine the lymph nodes? Here is why.

Arteries and veins carry blood to and from various parts of the body. Some fluid, called lymph, seeps out of these blood vessels, and is returned to the blood stream by a network of thin tubes called lymphatic ducts. It is this lymphatic fluid, or lymph, that helps the body wash away foreign particles or other debris that can collect in the spaces between cells.

Lymphatic ducts from the lungs come together in the mediastinum, the area between the lungs. There, the lymph is filtered through tiny bean-shaped organs called lymph nodes. Foreign particles (such as bacteria from an infection, or break-away cancer cells from a tumor in the lung) are trapped in the lymph nodes before they can enter the general circulation.

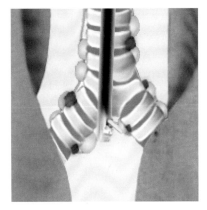

During the mediastinoscopy the surgeon will remove a few lymph nodes and send them to the pathologist for examination under the microscope, to determine whether cancer cells are present.

This information is extremely important for determining the stage of your cancer, and deciding whether you need additional therapy, such as chemotherapy.

AFTER YOUR OPERATION

When the surgery is completed, one or two tubes called chest tubes will be inserted through the skin of your chest and placed alongside the lung. The tubes will be attached to a suction device. The mild suction will help remove the fluid that accumulates at the site of surgery. More importantly, the suction will maintain the lung fully inflated as your chest wall moves as you breath. Before you go home, the tubes will be removed.

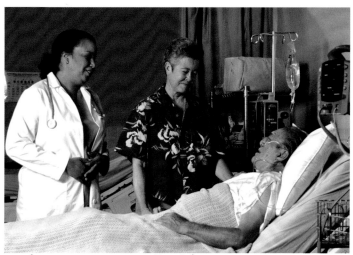

As you wake up, you will be wheeled into the recovery room. Special nurses will keep you under close observation as you drift in and out of your sleep for the next one to two hours. When you become more alert, you may be allowed a short visit by the person who accompanied you to the hospital.

From the recovery room you will be taken to your floor or to an intensive care unit for overnight stay.

Recovery

You will stay in the hospital for several days to recuperate. Right after surgery you will still have several tubes attached to your body. One will be an IV (or intravenous line) into your arm to replenish your fluids before you are able to ingest fluids by mouth.

You may have an *arterial line*. This is used to check your blood gases—and provide an indication of whether your remaining lung tissues is taking in enough oxygen.

You will probably also have one or two *chest tubes*, connected to a collection device and to suction. Chest tubes will remove any liquid or air that may leak from the surgical site into your chest cavity. This will help your lungs stay expanded.

Listening to the noise of the suction device may be irritating. Consider turning on some music, or using ear plugs if you need to.

The performance of the chest tubes will be checked periodically with chest X-rays.

Your goal should be to recover as much of your ability to breath as possible, as soon as possible.

The nurses and respiratory therapists will help you with breathing exercises. These may include forceful coughing to help re-expand the collapsed alveoli in your lungs.

You will be given a plastic tube called an *incentive spirometer.* You should use this every hour for at least ten breaths. This will help promote cough and expand your lungs.

It is very important that you do all of your lung exercises. They are meant to keep any complications, such as pneumonia, from developing.

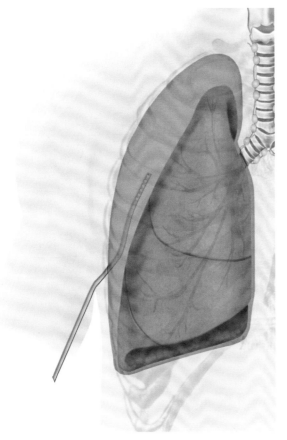

A chest tube will be connected to suction to expand your lung.

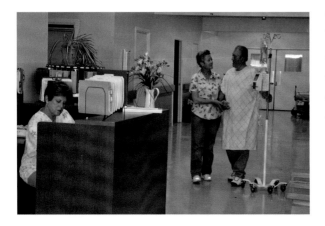

The staff will get you moving as soon as possible, to prevent complications such as blood clots. At first you might find it difficult to get out of bed, but each time you do, you will feel stronger. You might even look forward to a stroll with your loved one.

Pain Management

You will almost certainly have pain for the first few days after your operation. A lot of structures have been cut, and you cannot expect them to return to normal, pain-free, function immediately.

If you are in pain, it is important to tell the nurse or doctor as soon as possible. With your input, they will be able to find the right type and dose of pain medication for you.

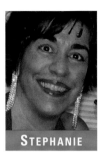

STEPHANIE

I am not a couch potato! I am active, type A, always on the go. And yet I couldn't sit up, I couldn't get out of bed. It took eight weeks before I could start to function semi normally.

While discomfort is to be expected, moderate to severe pain must be controlled—and not just for your comfort: If you are in pain, you will not be able to take the deep breaths, and to do your breathing exercises, that are so important to recovering your lung function. It is important that you are as comfortable as possible so that you can breathe properly and lower your risk of chest infection.

Pain medication works best when taken regularly, so don't suffer in silence. No matter how stoic you are, during recovery your motto should be "Pain? No gain," not the other way around.

Rarely, some people find they have pain that starts a few weeks or months after their operation. This is usually due to the fact that nerve endings that have been unavoidably damaged during the operation, have now started to grow back. This pain will go away when the nerve endings have recovered.

If you have any pain after your operation, do see your surgeon to find out what is causing the pain. If it cannot be managed easily, a referral to a pain specialist will almost certainly help.

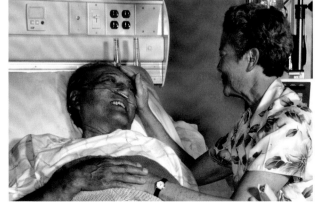

GOING HOME

You will probably be ready to go home about three to five days after your operation. If you live alone, or think that you will have difficulty managing, let the nurses know, so plans can be made to help you when you go home.

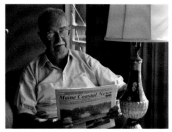

If you feel tired, rest.

Once you're home, you'll probably feel more tired than usual for a while. Don't be discouraged. You've just been through general anesthesia and major surgery, and fatigue is to be expected.

Take sponge baths for a few days after surgery until your incision starts to heal. Don't shower until your surgeon tells you that it is alright to get the incision wet. When you do shower, treat the skin gently and pat, rather than rub, the incision.

WOUND CARE

• You may be allowed to take a shower 48 hours after you go home. When you do shower, make sure that someone helps you remove the entire bandage.

• Fingertip-wash the incision area with a mild soap. Rinse the area with warm water and pat dry with a dry clean towel.

• You may apply an antibiotic ointment to the wound.

• Keep the dressing clean and dry. If the wound leaks, or the dressing becomes wet, change it immediately.

• You may leave the wound undressed, or use a piece of gauze loosely held with paper tape.

• If you run a fever, or if the wound becomes red, inflamed or leaks puss, please notify your surgeon at once.

ALI

My insurance covered renting a hospital style bed for my downstairs, so I wouldn't have to climb stairs. In three weeks, I recovered enough to drive myself to chemo.

It is important to begin an exercise routine to regain your strength and flexibility. Check with your doctor or physical therapist about exercise before you leave the hospital. It is important to start slowly and not overdo it. Many hospitals have post-operative respiratory and physical rehabilitation programs that you can attend as an outpatient. Walking around the house and then around your neighborhood is the best exercise to do on your own.

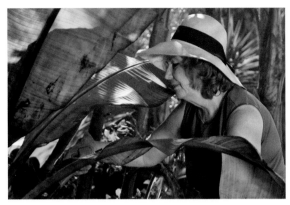

Resume work only when you feel ready.

Your doctor will tell you when you can start driving again. Usually it is about four to six weeks after a thoracotomy or two to three weeks after VATS. Some auto insurance companies also specify that you should not drive for a certain amount of time after chest surgery, so it is worth checking with your agent.

LUNG SURGERY RISKS

Lung surgery carries some of the same risks as other surgical procedures: bleeding, wound infection, and poor healing.

But there are additional risks such as an air leak in your lung that does not close, infection in the pleura (empyema), cardiac arrhythmias and other heart problems.

In addition, injury to your breathing muscles and ribs will make breathing painful for some time after surgery. This may decrease your ability to take deep, healthy breaths, and lead to pneumonia.

Your surgeon will review the risks with you before you sign the informed consent form.

•••

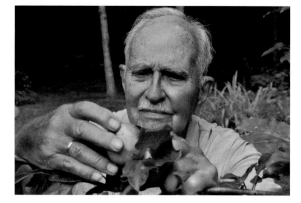

THE BENEFITS

Anticipating lung surgery is frightening. Recovering from lung surgery may be painful. But keep one thing in mind. In many cases of lung cancer, surgery offers you an important benefit that is well worth all the drawbacks: the best chance of a complete cure.

CHAPTER 6

RADIATION THERAPY

WHAT IS RADIATION THERAPY?

Radiation therapy (also called radiotherapy) uses high-energy X-rays to kill cancer cells. The treatment works by using the radiation to damage the genetic material, or DNA, within the cells, making it more difficult for them to divide. Both normal cells and cancer cells are affected, but normal cells can recover quickly, while the abnormal, rapidly dividing cancer cells, are permanently damaged.

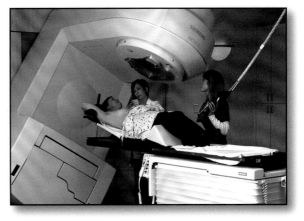

Radiation therapy can play many different roles in various stages of lung cancer – both NSCLC and SCLC.

The goals of the treatment will vary with the type and stage of cancer. Radiation can be used to attempt a cure, prevent the spread or manage symptoms.

Radiation therapy for lung cancer is generally administered by a complex device, called a linear accelerator, or linac machine, that aims a beam of radiation at the cancer area. This is called external beam radiation therapy, or EBRT.

In certain situations of lung cancer treatment, radiation therapy can be given by tiny radioactive seeds placed into or near the tumor. This is called internal radiation therapy or brachytherapy.

Let's start by looking at EBRT in detail.

EXTERNAL BEAM RADIATION THERAPY

External beam radiation therapy is the oldest and most common type o
radiation therapy.

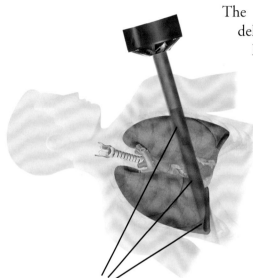

The goal of any successful course of radiation therapy is t
deliver the maximal dose of radiation to the cancer, with th
least damage to the surrounding normal tissues.

In years past, this was a challenging task. Here is why.

Imagine a lump the size of a grape, deep inside th
body – in the lung for example. If one were to aim
a single, stationary beam of radiation at that lump
one would eventually destroy the lump
Unfortunately, one would also destroy a tunnel o
normal tissue that the beam has to pass on the way to
and beyond the lump. Very likely, the damage migh
involve other vital organs, such as heart or liver. The
side effects of such treatment would be unacceptable.

Tissue damaged by single beam

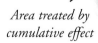

Now, imagine that you aim four beams, each
only one quarter as strong as the original,
from four different directions, all converg-
ing on the deep lump, like searchlights on
a fugitive. You have inflicted only one
quarter of the damage along each of the
four different pathways, but the lump still
received a full dose of radiation. Partially
damaged healthy tissue will recover. The fully
irradiated lump will not.

*Area treated by
cumulative effect*

The technology to achieve such precise control is
becoming more and more sophisticated every year.

Today's radiation therapy uses multiple radiation beams generated by a machine called a linear accelerator, or linac. The head of the device rotates around the patient, aiming beams of radiation from different angles. The impact on healthy tissue is diminished by being spread over a large volume. The effect on the target area, where the beams intersect, is increased.

A more refined form of this multi-beam approach is called 3-dimensional conformal radiotherapy (3D-CRT). This approach combines multiple radiation beams that are actually tailored to just the precise shape needed to radiate the cancerous area.

An improvement in radiotherapy is *intensity modulated radiation therapy*, or IMRT. Each beam is shaped in such a way that it will irradiate only the cancerous field, no matter what shape it appears from that particular angle.

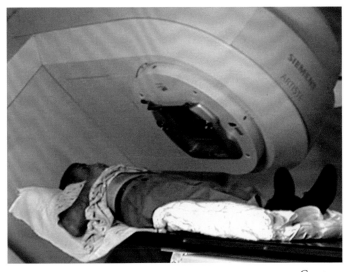

Courtesy
Siemens Medical Systems

Stereotactic body radiation therapy (**SBRT**) is similar to 3D-CRT, but it is more precise. Tiny metal seeds implanted into the tumor area are used as becons that enable the machinery to track the movement of the tumor during breathing. This makes it possible to deliver the radiation with much greater precision, while sparing the adjacent tissues.

Usually only three to five treatments are needed to complete the entire course. Because of the high doses used, SBRT is not for everyone.

Stereotactic radiosurgery (**SRS**) is a non-surgical radiation therapy used to treat small tumors. It can deliver precisely-targeted radiation in fewer high-dose treatments than traditional therapy, which can help preserve healthy tissue. When SRS is used to treat body tumors, it's called stereotactic body radiotherapy (SBRT).

Proton Beam Treatment

Another form of therapy utilizes a beam of protons. Unlike photon-based radiation therapy, which delivers the dose throughout the course of the beam path, proton therapy deposits the energy at a specific depth. This property gives protons a better dose distribution, thus limiting the damage to nearby critical structures.

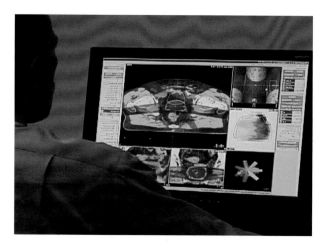

Treatment Planning

Needless to say, any highly sophisticated treatment process requires sophisticated planning and calculations, carefully tailored to each case. And radiotherapy is no exception.

Before external radiation begins, your radiation oncologist will work with highly skilled radiation therapy specialists to plan your treatment.

Using a CT scanner, the team will create a roadmap showing the tumor and surrounding tissues in three dimensions. Then, with the aid of powerful computers, multiple radiation beams will be calculated and shaped to the contour of the area to be treated.

The radiation therapist will mark your body with tiny tattoos to act as guides in aligning the radiation beam during treatments. Sometimes a special plaster mold will be fabricated for you to ensure consistent positioning.

TOMMA

They gave me treatments from two sides of the chest. I went in Monday through Friday. The commute was actually longer than the treatments.

Some of the more advanced linacs actually have a built-in CT scanner, allowing the treatment beams to be adjusted for every one of the many sessions that you will have during the course of treatment.

Once the planning is completed, the treatments can begin.

How Treatment is Given

Radiation treatments are administered by a radiation therapist in accordance with the plan developed for you by the team. Typically, you will arrive at the facility at the appointed time each day. You may want to bring a friend for moral support, at least during the first session or two. You may also want to bring an iPod or a book in case you have to wait.

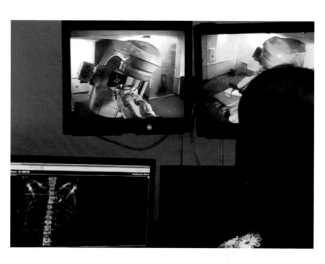

The first treatment after the planning session will take longers, in order to make sure the position matches the angles that were worked out during simulation.

Treatments are given in a room that has thick concrete walls and lead-lined doors, to protect those who are outside the treatment area from radiation.

Your radiation therapist will keep you in sight at all times.

The device used to deliver radiation, the linear accelerator is large and complex. At first the whole set up may be intimidating. But don't be alarmed. A TV monitor lets the staff keep you in sight at all times, and you and the staff can communicate with one another via intercom.

The radiation therapists will adjust the position of the machine according to the previously determined settings, using intersecting laser beams as guides. Then the therapists will step out of the room. During the actual exposure you must remain as still as possible. The unit will reposition itself several times to change the angle of the beam. Each exposure lasts only a few minutes. The best part is that you won't feel anything.

Daily trips to the radiation therapy facility may conflict with your daily routine or work requirements. If you have to miss a session or two, discuss the situation with your doctor or nurse. You can make up the days at the end, but the effectiveness of the treatment depends on having as few delays as possible.

KAY

My doctor told me, "NED." No evidence of disease. The tumor was dead, thanks to SBRT, and to CyberKnife. I felt blessed.

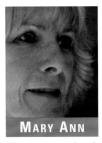

MARY ANN

Chemo seemed to be OK. I knew something toxic was going into me. But radiation… it scared me. You don't see it, you don't hear it. You don't know what is really going on… Totally irrational fear.

Duration of Treatment

The length of your treatment depends on the goal: a long series to completely eliminate a small tumor, or one or two shots to shrink a blockage.

A full course of treatment may involve daily treatment sessions, Monday through Friday with rest on weekends, for five to seven weeks.

The same full dose of radiation can sometimes be given in much larger, but fewer doses, or fractions: for example twice a day for five days saving you the repetitive daily trips to the hospital.

When the goal of radiotherapy is to simply shrink the tumor enough to relive symptoms, such as difficulty breathing, the course of treatment may be much shorter—perhaps only a few sessions.

SIDE EFFECTS OF EXTERNAL BEAM RADIATION THERAPY

Radiation therapy is a safe, proven treatment, but it does have a few unwanted side effects. Most of them are due to the fact that the radiation beam affects normal tissues around the tumor area—most importantly, the lung, heart and esophagus.

The side effects that you may develop depend on the type and timing of the treatment you receive. If you have dozens of sessions over several weeks, your side effects will be different from what you can expect if you only had one or two doses.

Side effects usually develop slowly, last for a few weeks after your treatment has ended, and then gradually disappear.

A small number of people have long term side effects, which develop up to two years after the treatment has ended.

The most common side effects include fatigue, skin changes, esophageal symptoms, such as sore throat and trouble swallowing, cough due to irritation to air passages, hair loss in the treated area, and chest pain.

Fatigue

Fatigue is often due to stress related to your illness, daily trips for treatment, and the effects of radiation on normal cells. Most people begin to feel tired after a few weeks of radiation therapy, and the fatigue will probably increase until the end of treatment. You can help yourself by not trying to do too much. If you feel tired, limit your activities, use your leisure time in a restful way, and try to get more sleep at night. Light exercise will actually decrease your fatigue, but pace yourself.

If you continue working a full-time job while undergoing radiation therapy, talk with your employer about adjusting your work schedule, or try working at home for a period of time.

Skin Changes

One of the effects of radiation therapy may mimic sunburn. Your skin may become very red, itchy or become tan or darkened. One of the most important things you can do during therapy is to follow the advice of the radiation nurse to prevent your skin from breaking down or blistering. The nurse will advise you to moisturize the skin by using pure aloe gel or Aquaphor. Whichever one works best for you should be applied two-three times a day but should not be on your skin when you come in for treatment.

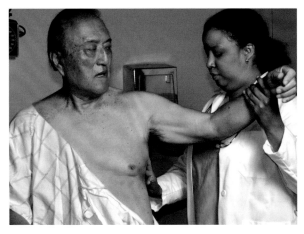

Sore throat and trouble swallowing

Your throat may become sore about two to three weeks into your treatment as a result of the effect of radiation on your esophagus. This is called esophagitis. You may feel that you have a lump in your throat or burning in your chest. You may also experience trouble swallowing.

There are different ways to manage these symptoms, including eating moist, soft foods such as cooked cereal, mashed potatoes or pudding. You may find it helpful to avoid excessively hot, spicy or dry foods.

QUESTIONS TO ASK
YOUR DOCTOR:

• Why do I need radiation therapy?

• How will I evaluate the effectiveness of the treatments?

• Can I continue my usual work or exercise schedule?

• Can I miss a few treatments?

• Can I arrange to be treated elsewhere if I am traveling?

• What side effects, if they occur, should I report immediately?

Your physician or nurse can advise you on other ways to relieve your symptoms and prescribe anaesthetic mouthwashes and antacids.

Cough

Cough is quite common during or after radiotherapy for lung cancer. The cough should pass when the treatment is over. Do tell your doctor if you feel feverish, because this might be the sign of an infection, and you may need antibiotics.

Hair loss

You will lose hair in the area being treated. The hair usually grows back within a few months, but it can be patchy.

Chest pain

You may experience chest pain if you are on one of the accelerated treatments, consisting of only one or two fractions. The pain can be managed with analgesics.

Long-term side effects

Long-term side effects may develop many months after your treatment. Most of them will be due to scar tissue formation, also referred to as fibrosis, caused by the development of fibrous tissue. Your symptoms may include shortness of breath due to loss of elasticity in the airways, or difficulty swallowing due to narrowing of the esophagus.

OTHER USES FOR RADIATION THERAPY

Radiation therapy is also used to relieve symptoms in cases when the disease cannot be cured. For example, if a tumor that cannot be removed surgically begins to obstruct an airway, radiation therapy can be used to shrink the tumor and reopen the passage. In other cases, tumors may have spread to other parts of the body. These metastases may sometimes cause pain. By treating them with a few sessions of radiation therapy, the metastases can be shrunk, and the pain relieved. This type of radiation therapy is called palliative.

INTERNAL RADIATION THERAPY - BRACHYTHERAPY

In some cases the most effective way to deliver radiation therapy may not be from outside your body, but from inside. This is done with radioactive pellets – or a radioactive source – placed into, or near the tumor. This method is called internal radiation therapy, or brachytherapy.

Unlike external beam radiation therapy, internal radiation therapy is not used as the main treatment to cure lung cancer. Instead, IRT is most effective for treating small areas. For example, to shrink a tumor that is blocking an airway, so you can breathe better.

The course of treatment begins with a planning session. This generally involves a CT scan of the area to verify the exact location of the tumor, and to determine the number and exact location of radioactive pellets to be used.

You will then have a bronchoscopy: a special tube, equipped with a viewing device, will be inserted through your nose or mouth and passed all the way to the location of the tumor.

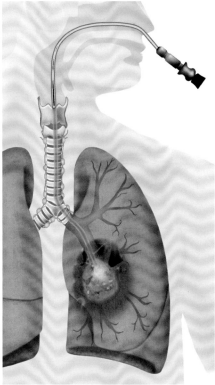

Using the bronchoscope for guidance, a hollow tube, called a catheter, will be threaded into the area.

Finally, a number of tiny radioactive pellets will be passed down the tube and left behind in the lung. The tube and the bronchoscope will be withdrawn, and you will be released to go home.

In some cases the seeds are implanted right after lung surgery. Whatever method is used, over the period of a few days, the pellets will release enough radiation to treat the target area, killing the cancerous cells. Eventually the pellets will lose their radioactivity and become entirely harmless.

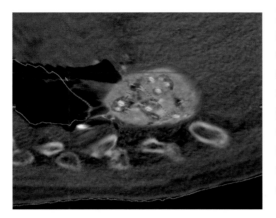

In another technique, instead of radioactive pellets being left behind, the radiation oncologist may use the catheter to place a tiny radioactive source next to, or within, the tumor. The source will remain in place for a few minutes to deliver the necessary dose of radiation. Both the radioactive source and the tube will then be removed. The treatment may be repeated again if needed.

ROLE OF RADIATION THERAPY

How may radiation therapy, either internal or external, fit into your treatment plan?

If you have early stage NSCLC, the best option for complete removal of the tumor – and a cure – is surgery. But if your overall health would make surgery risky, radiation therapy may be an excellent, low risk alternative.

A full course of radiation treatments can be effective in eliminating a small tumor and achieving a cure. This type of treatment may be referred to as radical radiotherapy. Radical radiotherapy may be given with daily sessions over four to seven weeks, or with three daily sessions over three weeks.

In many cases a combination of radiation therapy and chemotherapy (chemoradiation) is used to treat lung cancer either before or after surgery. Although this treatment is difficult on the patient, it can be very effective and is used for curative intent.

Radiation therapy may also be your best choice if the cancer is in a location that is difficult to reach surgically without damage to other organs. For example, cancers that grow right at the top of the lung can be very close to the nerves that supply the arm and this can make them very difficult to operate on.

TOMMA

Toward the end of the treatment, the fatigue became cumulative. So I had to be driven the last month. But I enjoyed the one on one time with my friends.

Radiation therapy can also sometimes play a role in SCLC treatment. Small cell lung cancer responds very well to radiation therapy. Your medical team may suggest radiation therapy after or together with chemotherapy to help prevent a recurrence after the tumor has been removed surgically.

Finally, radiation therapy can also be used prophylactically – in other words, to prevent the cancer from spreading. This is particularly effective in SCLC, which tends to metastacize to the brain. If your cancer responded well to chemotherapy, your medical team will recommend that you have a short course of radiation to the head. This is called *prophylactic cranial irradiation*, or simply PCI. PCI will greatly decrease the chance of cancer spread to your brain.

•••

THE BENEFITS

Radiation therapy may be intimidating and inconvenient. But remember, in many cases, it may be the most effective tool for managing your disease, with less impact on your ability to pursue your daily activities.

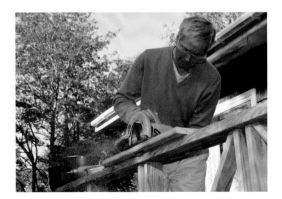

CHAPTER 7

CHEMOTHERAPY

LOCAL VS. SYSTEMIC TREATMENT

The goal of any cancer treatment is to completely eliminate every single cancer cell from the body. This is generally attempted by fighting the cancer in two different ways: with local treatment and with systemic treatment.

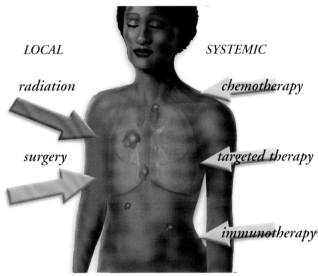

Local therapies include *surgery* and *radiation*. Surgery removes the tumor from the body. Radiation targets any cancer cells that might have been left behind after the tumor was removed. Both of these work on the tumor itself. Both were discussed in previous chapters.

Local therapies work in the lung area only
Systemic therapies work on the entire body

Systemic therapies kill cancer cells anywhere in the body, including those cells that might have broken off the tumor and traveled to other organs. Systemic therapies can be in the form of *chemotherapy* (drugs that kill cancer cells), *targeted therapy* or *immunotherapy* (drugs that help your body fight off cancer) or a combination of these.

We will talk about chemotherapy in this chapter, and about targeted therapy in the next chapter.

QUESTIONS TO ASK
YOUR DOCTOR:

- **Do I need chemotherapy? Why?**

- **What drugs do you recommend?**

- **What are the benefits and risks of chemotherapy?**

- **How successful is this treatment for the type of cancer I have?**

- **How will you evaluate the effectiveness of the treatments?**

- **What side effects will I experience?**

- **Can I work while I'm having chemotherapy?**

- **Can I travel between treatments (short business or pleasure trips)?**

- **What other limitations can I expect?**

WHAT IS CHEMOTHERAPY?

Chemotherapy is the use of cytotoxic (cell-killing) drugs that either kill cancer cells or prevent them from growing and dividing. One or, usually, several different drugs are given in order to disrupt the cell growth cycle. Chemotherapy is a versatile tool and can be used in different ways:

Neoadjuvant chemotherapy is chemotherapy that is used before surgery or radiation therapy, in order to shrink a tumor, and improve the results of the primary treatment.

Adjuvant chemotherapy is used as an addition to the local treatment to decrease the chances of cancer spread.

Palliative chemotherapy is given to relieve symptoms of the cancer (such as pain), without the expectation of curing the disease. Palliative care is a comfort measure.

HOW CHEMOTHERAPY WORKS

Cells go through several steps in the process of cell division. First, the genetic material (DNA) forms strands called chromosomes. Then the chromosomes divide into two sets, and the cell enlarges. Finally the cell splits into two identical cells, each with its own set of DNA. This cycle repeats itself.

Chemotherapy drugs interfere with various parts of this cycle, making it difficult for the cells to reproduce and repair themselves. Often several different drugs are used simultaneously in order to target different parts of the cycle and achieve the best result.

DO YOU NEED CHEMOTHERAPY?

Many patients are reluctant to face chemotherapy, because they still have the old misconception that chemotherapy is something that makes you deathly ill, or makes your hair fall out.

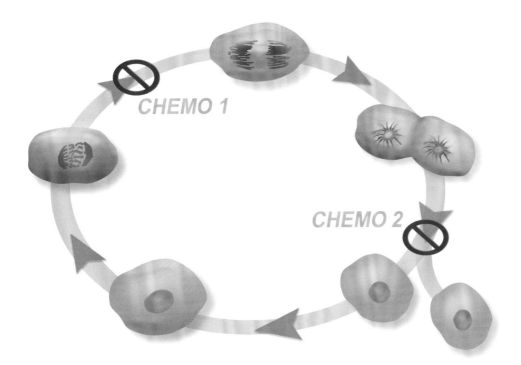

Different chemotherapy drugs disrupts different parts of the cell division cycle

Much has changed in recent years. Today there are very effective drugs that can greatly reduce—and sometimes eliminate—the side effects of chemotherapy, making the experience much more tolerable than it was in the past.

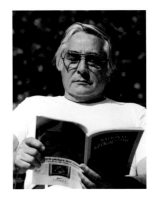

Do you personally need chemotherapy? The chemotherapy decision will depend on a variety of factors related to your cancer, your health and your mindset.

New developments in genetic testing are being used to predict whether chemotherapy will help you, and to find the most effective drugs for your particular case.

THE CHEMOTHERAPY DECISION DEPENDS ON:

• Your cancer, focusing on such features as size, cell type, grade, and rate of growth.

• Your individual profile, considering age, health, tumor location, and lymph node involvement.

• Stage of your disease, which is determined by tumor size, tumor cell invasion, node involvement, and spread to other organs.

• Risk/benefit assessment, taking in consideration the possible side effects and the expected long term results.

Here is a look at where chemotherapy may be used to treat lung cancer.

SCLC

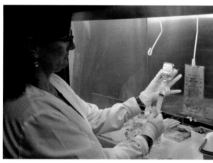

If you have SCLC, chemotherapy will probably be your best treatment choice. For two reasons:

• SCLC tumors respond very well to chemotherapy.

• SCLC tumors tend to have microscopic spread when they are first diagnosed. Spread that is invisible cannot be treated surgically.

In some cases, very early, small SCLC tumors might be treated with surgery, but your physician will suggest additional treatment with chemotherapy (adjuvant therapy) to target the microscopic clusters of cancer cells that probably have spread throughout the body.

The most commonly used chemotherapy combination for small cell cancers is cisplatin and etoposide. But there are many other combinations, including carboplatin with etoposide, and cyclophosphamide with doxorubicin and vincristine.

NSCLC

Chemotherapy is also used in NSCLC:

It can be used before surgery or radiation therapy to shrink the tumor (neoadjuvant therapy).

Or it can be used after surgery or radiation to kill any cancer cells that may remain, and lower the risk of cancer recurrence (adjuvant chemotherapy).

Chemotherapy will not cure advanced-stage lung cancer, but it can relieve some symptoms and may slow cancer growth.

Your physicians will help you evaluate objectively the expected advantages and disadvantages of chemotherapy.

In discussing your options with your medical team, remember that chemotherapy, despite the side effects, offers you the benefits of being one of the most powerful tools for fighting lung cancer available today.

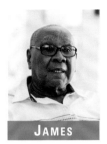

JAMES

Don't eat your favorite food when you are on chemo, because you will develop an aversion reaction to it. And you don't want to not ever eat chocolate again, do you?

HOW CHEMOTHERAPY IS GIVEN

Some chemotherapy drugs come in pill form, and you take them at home, just as you would any other pill. Others are given by injection into a vein (called intravenous or IV chemo). These injections can be given in a private doctor's office, in a hospital, or in a cancer center.

Chemo is given in cycles. For example, one dose every three to four weeks, with rest on the fourth week. The rest periods allows the normal cells in your body to recover between treatments. The full course of therapy takes four to six month-long cycles, but could be longer or shorter depending on your particular case. You will probably start chemotherapy within six weeks after surgery.

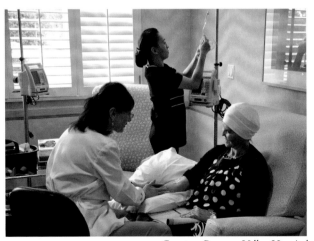

Courtesy Pomona Valley Hospital

Chemotherapy is usually given by intravenous injection in outpatient centers

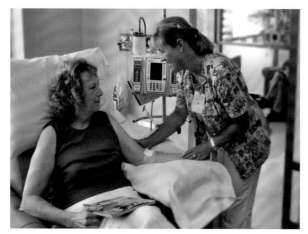

Courtesy St. Joseph Hospital of Orange

Your experience with chemotherapy will depend on several things, including whether you are taking oral or IV chemotherapy.

If you are on intravenous therapy, you will receive the injections in an oncologist's office, or at an outpatient treatment center. Before you get the scheduled dose of chemotherapy, the nurse will draw your blood to check whether the treatment has affected the blood-producing cells in your bone marrow, or the function of your liver or other organs. If your blood counts are too low, your oncologist may decide to lower the dose of chemo, or delay the treatment.

If your results are acceptable, the nurse will take you to the treatment area and start the IV (intravenous line) through which the drug will be injected.

If your veins are easy to reach, this will take a few seconds, and feel like a pinprick. Then the drug will be injected. Some drugs are given as a rapid injection, others are dripped in slowly, over a longer period—sometimes up to three hours. Generally you won't feel any discomfort.

Ports

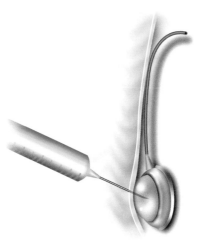

Sometimes veins are thin, damaged, or covered by a layer of fat, making them difficult to reach. A few IV chemo drugs can be very irritating to the vein, and can damage it. In such cases your physician may recommend that an infusion port be installed under your skin. These devices make it easier to administer your medications with the least damage to your veins, and can also be used for drawing blood, thus avoiding needle sticks during clinic visits.

A port consists of a tube (catheter), attached to a dome-shaped part. The device is surgically implanted under the skin, with the dome placed in the chest or arm, where it will be easily accessible for injections through a needle, but will not interfere with your activities. The catheter is threaded into a large vein, where rapid blood flow will dilute the drug, and keep it from damaging the lining of the vein. Since the port is completely covered by skin, you can shower, swim and exercise freely. The port will be removed after your treatment ends.

SIDE EFFECTS OF CHEMOTHERAPY

Anti-cancer drugs work by preventing cells from growing and dividing. The effect is strongest on cancer cells, but normal tissues can be affected, too, particularly those where the cells are growing rapidly, such as hair, intestinal tract, and bone marrow. The most common side effects are related to these organs, and include nausea, fatigue, menopausal symptoms and hair loss. The side effects will vary with the drug used, and with your own tolerance to it.

> **STEPHANIE:** I thought I understood chemo from watching my husband go through it. But you really don't understand till you go through it. On the bad days I would just go to my room and stay in bed. I called them my chemo coma days. Then you start getting better, then it was time for the next treatment. But somehow you just get through it.

While it is important to be prepared for possible side effects of chemotherapy, it is equally important not to assume that you will have all, many, or even a few of them. Also keep in mind that most side effects are temporary and go away when treatment ends. And many side effects can be treated or even prevented.

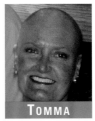

TOMMA

My nurse said, you will have one bad day each cycle. She was right. I would get my injections on Friday, and Monday I couldn't get out of bed. But I still went to work all the other days. I am stubborn that way...

Bone marrow produces...

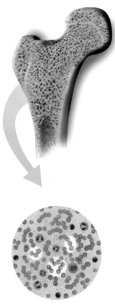

red blood cells,

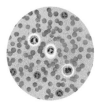

white blood cells,

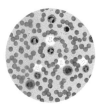

and platelets.

Nausea

Today, thanks to powerful antiemetic drugs, nausea is much less common than in years past. Discuss your symptoms with your healthcare professionals, and make sure that you are receiving the best anti-nausea medication for your particular needs.

Fatigue

Chemotherapy can make you feel tired, especially on the first day after each treatment. This fatigue is not like the one after a hard day's work. It is much more general, and may not get better with rest.

Many patients find that given some flexibility they can keep a fairly normal level of activity. If you feel totally unable to function at a reasonable level, tell your oncologist about it. Your drug dose may need to be readjusted. In addition, your physician may recommend medications to help your body rebuild red blood cells, and raise your energy level. Your fatigue may be also caused by lack of sleep, by pain, or by poor food intake.

Bone Marrow Suppression

Bone marrow cells, which produce red blood cells, white blood cells, and platelets for your blood, are particularly affected by chemotherapy, and may lose some, or all, of their function, leading to lower blood cell counts.

Red blood cells (RBC's) carry oxygen to all cells in your body. The normal value for red cell oxygen carrying capacity, is 12 to 14 mgHb. A low red blood cell count, called anemia, may give you fatigue, a pale skin, shortness of breath, dizziness, or a rapid heart beat.

White blood cells (WBC's) help fight infection. A normal WBC count is in the 5,000-10,000 range. The most important type of WBCs for fighting infection are called neutrophils. When your WBC counts get low you are at a high risk for infection and your cancer care team may talk to you about special precautions you should take until your WBC count recovers.

Platelets help the blood clot. A low platelet count, below 100,000, can lead to dangerous bleeding. The signs you may notice are easy bruising, excessive bleeding from wounds, or black stools——an indication of bleeding into the stomach or intestine.

To anticipate all these potentially serious complications, your healthcare team will check your blood counts often. Your chemotherapy dose will be adjusted to achieve the maximum effect on the tumor cells, without dangerously impairing the ability of the bone marrow to produce blood cells in sufficient quantities.

If your bone marrow becomes suppressed, and is not making enough blood cells, your doctor may add medications to your treatment, to stimulate your bone marrow to produce more blood cells. You may also have platelet or whole blood transfusions.

Infections

When your white blood cell count is low, your body may not be able to fight off infections, even if you take extra care. Most infections come from bacteria normally found on the skin, in the intestines, and in the genital tract.

Be alert to signs that you might have an infection, and report them to your doctor right away. This is especially important when your white blood cell count is low. If you have a fever, don't use aspirin, acetaminophen (Tylenol), or any other medicine to bring your temperature down without first checking with your doctor.

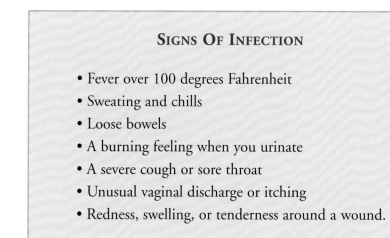

SIGNS OF INFECTION

- Fever over 100 degrees Fahrenheit
- Sweating and chills
- Loose bowels
- A burning feeling when you urinate
- A severe cough or sore throat
- Unusual vaginal discharge or itching
- Redness, swelling, or tenderness around a wound.

STEPHANIE

Hair loss... My message to women, Don't be vain! It is the least of your problems. It will grow back.

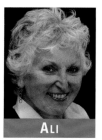

ALI

I didn't have nausea, but the platinum based chemo drug they put me on had bad side effects. Really bad taste in my mouth from silverware, or even anything packed in metal. I once threw away a perfectly good can of tuna, because it tasted foul. Turned out it was the chemo. But to this day I can't eat tuna.

QUESTIONS TO ASK
YOUR DOCTOR:

- **Will my chemo be given IV or in pill form?**

- **How will I know if the pills are working?**

- **What side effects can I expect?**

PREVENTING INFECTIONS

- Wash your hands often during the day.

- Clean your rectal area after each bowel movement.

- Avoid people with diseases, but feel free to go out.

- Don't cut or tear the cuticles off your nails.

- Be careful not to cut or nick yourself.

- Use an electric shaver instead of a razor to prevent cuts.

- Use a soft toothbrush that won't hurt your gums.

- Don't squeeze or scratch pimples.

- Take a warm bath, shower, or sponge bath every day.

- Clean cuts right away with warm water and an antiseptic.

- Wear protective gloves when gardening or cleaning up.

- Check with your doctor before getting immunizations.

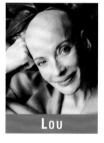

LOU

True to form, after about five weeks into the chemo, my hair started coming out so much that I felt like a dandelion blowing in the wind.

Raising your white cell count (WBC) will help you fight off infections. An extremely low white blood count can delay your chemotherapy, or keep you from receiving your full dose—and its benefits. Your oncologist may recommend the use of a white cell booster or growth factor such as Neupogen or Neulasta. Restoring your bone marrow function may make the difference between completing a full course of chemotherapy, or quitting prematurely.

OTHER SIDE EFFECTS

Some of the other side effects of chemotherapy may include mouth sores, loss of appetite, intestinal problems, hair loss, and tingling of fingers and toes.

If you develop sores in your mouth, be sure to contact your doctor or nurse right away. Mouth sores can make it hard to eat, can be very painful, and can lead to infection. You may need medical treatment to keep the sores from getting worse.

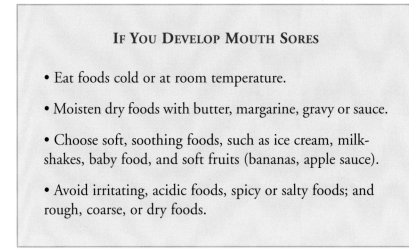

IF YOU DEVELOP MOUTH SORES

• Eat foods cold or at room temperature.

• Moisten dry foods with butter, margarine, gravy or sauce.

• Choose soft, soothing foods, such as ice cream, milk-shakes, baby food, and soft fruits (bananas, apple sauce).

• Avoid irritating, acidic foods, spicy or salty foods; and rough, coarse, or dry foods.

ALI

Chemo was OK because I had anti-nausea drugs. Now, mind you they will try to give you the cheapest anti-nausea. But if that doesn't work for you, demand the best. You don't have to suffer. The drugs are available.

When chemotherapy affects the lining of the intestine, the result may be diarrhea. Discuss the problem with your healthcare provider. There are things that will help correct the problem, such as eating smaller portions more often, and avoid high fiber foods.

Do not take any over-the-counter medications unless specifically recommended by your healthcare provider.

TOMMA

My hair did fall out. But you have to just expect it, and accept it. I did the proactive thing – I picked out a wig ahead of time. Still that first look in the mirror shakes you up a little...

Hair loss is not harmful, but can be very upsetting. If hair loss does occur, it most often begins within two weeks of the start of treatment and gets worse at one to two months. Be aware that you can lose all the hair on your body—including eyebrows, eyelashes, and pubic hair. The hair grows back after treatment, though it may be a different texture or color.

> LOU : I went out with the Mohawk a couple of times and had fun scaring small children. And as far as being bald goes, here is a little-known secret: being bald feels AMAZING. I now love having all the windows down when I drive. My hair doesn't get stuck to my lipstick when I turn my head in a breeze. I can get ready in eleven minutes flat. And your skull can be a very funky-sounding percussive instrument when you get bored. Who knew?

QUESTIONS TO ASK YOUR DOCTOR:

- **How can I manage nausea?**

- **Will I be given medications to treat side effects?**

- **Can I take public transportation home after treatments?**

- **Can I take vitamins or herbs if I choose?**

There is one more side effect that you may experience: *chemo brain.* Chemo brain is a common term used by cancer survivors to describe thinking and memory problems that can occur after chemotherapy treatment. It's not clear that chemo brain is caused by chemotherapy, but it's clear that it can be frustrating and debilitating. Usually, the chemo brain feeling will improve with time.

•••

It is probably safe to say that you aren't looking forward to chemo. But as you go through this taxing treatment, remember one thing: Chemotherapy is one of the most effective tools we have for battling lung cancer.

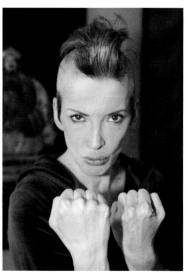

CHAPTER 8

TARGETED THERAPY & IMMUNOTHERAPY

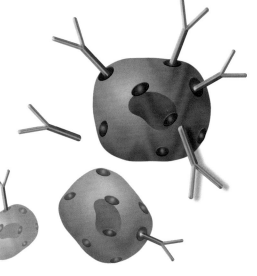

WHAT ARE TARGETED THERAPIES?

Chemotherapy drugs work by attacking all fast-growing cells in the body. Fortunately, this includes cancer cells. Unfortunately, it also includes the rapidly multiplying but normal cells of the gastrointestinal tract, bone marrow, skin, hair and other organs.

For a long time, scientists have been looking for new drugs that could tell the difference between normal and cancerous cells. Recently, this search has produced a number of breakthroughs.

Target therapy molecules home in on specific receptor sites on the surface of a lung cancer cell

Targeted therapy, is a promising approach to cancer treatment. As cancer cell tests have evolved, it became clear that no two cancers are alike. Many differ from each other in that their DNA has specific mutations that can be identified. As a result, it became possible to develop chemical agents that act specifically against the target mutation. Think of it as the difference between shooting with a wide-scatter shot gun, or a precisely aimed rifle.

For example, some cells have mutations in the Human Epidermal Growth Factor, or EGFR gene, a protein located on the surface of the cells helps them divide, enabling the tumor to grow. Drugs have been developed to specifically target mutant EGFR, making them more effective.

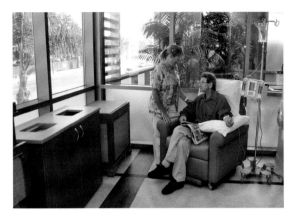

Courtesy
St. Joseph Hospital of Orange

Other drugs are used to target a certain mutation in the ALK gene present in non-small cell lung cancers.

As a result of this more precise approach, it becomes possible to use drugs that cause less unintended damage to healthy tissues — hence fewer side effects.

Your physician may recommend molecular testing to determine whether your tumor contains specific gene mutations, and whether you will benefit from targeted therapy.

Anti-neogenesis

Cancerous tumors create new blood vessels through a process called *angiogenesis.* The new blood vessels help cancer cells grow and spread.

Anti-angiogenesis drugs target the process that enables the growth of blood vessels. Without blood supply, the tumor is starved of the nutrients and oxygen it needs to grow and spread.

SIDE EFFECTS OF TARGETED THERAPIES

Even though the drugs designed for targeted therapy are focused on specific abnormal cells, they still affect normal cells, and cause unwanted side effects. The side effects depend on the drug and on the patient, and only your medical team can advise you on the risks and benefits in your particular case.

WHO CAN BENEFIT FROM TARGETED THERAPIES?

Presently, not every patient, and not every lung cancer case can be teated with targeted therapy. A sample of your tumor will be sent for a variety of tests, either right after the biopsy, or at a later date, to determine which, if any, targeted therapies could benefit you.

Scientists are searching for new markers that will help us develop additional, and better-focused targeted therapies. Ask your doctor to review the latest findings with you.

QUESTIONS TO ASK
YOUR DOCTOR:

- **Can my tumor be treated with targeted therapy?**

- **If not, why not?**

- **What drugs do you recommend?**

- **What side effects can I expect with this treatment?**

- **Will I be given medications to treat side effects?**

IMMUNOTHERAPY

Perhaps the most exciting developments—some scientists call them revolutionary advances—in the past two-to-five years have been in the area of *immunotherapy*, also called biotherapy.

The normally healthy human body has a potent self-defense mechanism that includes T cells designed to fend off attacks by foreign tissues, bacteria and viruses. Why not cancer cells?

The problem is that cancer cells often "trick" the immune system into accepting them as normal, or creating a camouflage effect that keeps the immune system from recognizing the threat.

For example, certain cancers have a surface protein called PD-L1. When the immune system attempts to attack, the cancer's PD-L1 protein orders the T cells to stand down. It does it by binding to another protein on the surface of the T cells, called PD-1, which acts as an "off switch," deactivating the T cells.

In a process called *check point inhibition* newly developed drugs prevent this binding, allowing the T cells to continue their attack.

Studies continue to evaluate the benefits of immunotherapy, and determine how it can be used instead of, or in conjunction with, traditional chemotherapy. But it is exciting to think that we are getting closer to learning how to harness our own bodily defenses in the fight against cancer.

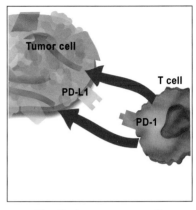

T cells destroy cancer cells.

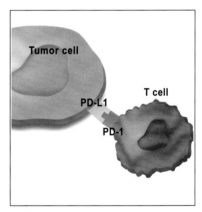

PD-L1 link inhibits T cells.

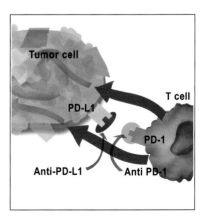

Anti-PD-L1 or Anti-PD-1 drugs can be used to prevent PD-L1 from binding to PD-1, making it impossible for the cancer cell to inhibit the T cell.

QUESTIONS TO ASK
YOUR DOCTOR:

- What are the benefits and risks of targeted therapy?

- How successful is this treatment for the type of cancer I have?

- How will you evaluate the effectiveness of the treatments?

- Can I work while I'm undergoing therapy?

- Can I travel between treatments (short business or pleasure trips)?

- What other limitations can I expect?

- What test should be ordered to see if I would benefit from immunotherapy?

GENE THERAPY

Other therapies include injecting cancer cells with special genes that make the tumor more receptive to the effects of anticancer drugs, or introducing the multi-drug resistant (MDR) gene into bone marrow to make stem cells more immune to the toxic side effects of anticancer drugs. It is a complicated area of research, and many questions remain unanswered. Talk to your cancer specialist about the implications of gene therapy.

•••

Looking toward the future, the new technologies offer new hope for effective treatment, for cure, and perhaps even prevention of lung cancer. Someday a new technology may even make conventional chemotherapy obsolete.

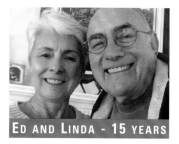

ED AND LINDA - 15 YEARS

After studying Ed's tumor they could tell the immunotherapy was working. So he is still on it. He is doing great and his attitude and willingness to live on never waivers.

CHAPTER 9

COMPLEMENTARY AND ALTERNATIVE THERAPIES

WHAT IS THE DIFFERENCE?

Conventional treatments for lung cancer—surgery, chemotherapy, radiation therapy and so on—are treatment methods that have been extensively tested by medical experts, and have proven their effectiveness. More than likely one or more of them will play a part in your treatment and recovery.

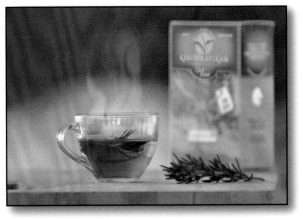

While researching your options, you may hear about other methods, such as special diets, acupuncture, new compounds, or new technologies. Some of these methods may deserve a place in your treatment plan. Others are just plain harmful.

It's extremely important that you understand the differences among the three different philosophies: conventional medicine, complementary therapies, and alternative therapies.

Conventional treatment is what is currently accepted as standard by reputable healthcare providers. It is based on decades of sound medical research, and represents the best that Western medicine has to offer today.

Don't worry, you will not be short-changing yourself by relying on conventional medicine. Although it is called "conventional" it does include the latest developments, leading-edge research, and the most advanced techniques.

Complementary treatments are what the name implies: a complement. In other words, an addition, to your treatment. Complementary treatments may or may not have been rigorously evaluated by scientific research. But over time they have been widely and successfully used to relieve side effects of cancer treatment, and to enhance the quality of life.

Alternative therapies are just that—different ways to do something, at the exclusion of conventional methods. Alternative therapies have no medically sound foundation, and no demonstrable value in prolonging or improving life. And they represent a dangerous temptation for those who may be skeptical about traditional medical treatment, or desperately seeking a cure.

Consult your healthcare team before trying any type of complementary or alternative therapy, to be sure it won't interfere with your medical treatment.

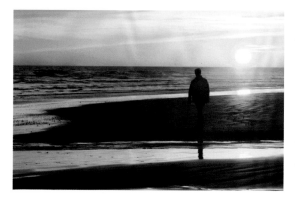

MIND-BODY CONNECTION

You understand how external therapies work. Surgery removes the tumor. Chemotherapy kills the cancer cells. But there is another form of therapy as well: the effect your own mind has on your body. Many complementary therapies are based on this age-old principle of mind-body connection: the state of the mind affects the health of the body.

How does this happen? During the cancer experience the nervous system is assaulted by stress, grief, fear and pain. And this can have a negative impact on the body: your energy levels, your ability to heal and your immune system may all be compromised. There is nothing mysterious about this. Scientists know that these effects are mediated by neurotransmitters—chemicals released by your brain.

Using a wide variety of approaches—such as meditation, visualization, physical activity, and spiritual support—may help you learn to cope with negative emotions, restore your emotional balance, and speed your recovery.

COMPLEMENTARY THERAPIES

There is a wide variety of complementary techniques, some based on principles adopted from other specialties (for example, relaxation), from Oriental medicine (acupuncture), from Indian medicine (yoga), or even from ancient Egyptian culture (aromatherapy). All of them have been used by cancer patients for a variety of purposes and with a variety of results. Whether they may fit into your treatment plan is up to you and your medical team.

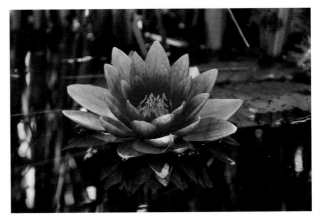

Meditation

Meditation attempts to quiet the busy mind by focusing it on the present moment. It may be as simple as listening to birds, or enjoying the feel of the breeze on your skin. There is no claim that meditation cures cancer, but studies have proven that it can reduce stress, pain and other uncomfortable side effects of cancer treatment.

Visualization

Focusing your mind on an image of natural beauty, or creating a peaceful scene in your imagination can help reduce stress, relieve pain, and enhance the immune system.

Yoga

Yoga, a practice of posturing and breathing, increases your range of motion, flexibility, strength, and leads to relaxation and a sense of well being. Yoga can be practiced as a way to clear the mind through meditation and breathing. Most postures can be modified to fit any person's physical ability.

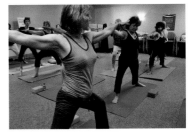

Massage

Rubbing, kneading and stroking your muscles and joints can help relieve tension, stress, anxiety, pain, and encourage relaxation. It is important to find a massage therapist specializing in treating cancer patients.

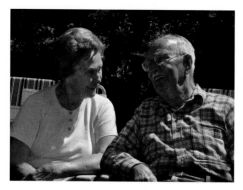

Humor and Laughter

Laughter can stimulate endorphins—chemicals that act like opiates in the brain. You might find humor and laughter emotionally healing.

In addition, giving yourself time not to think about your cancer can have a wonderfully invigorating effect. Treat yourself to a comedy, read a joke book, or just allow yourself a moment of levity. It may prove a welcome addition to your daily routine.

Acupuncture

QUESTIONS TO ASK YOUR DOCTOR:

How can I be certified to receive medical marijuana?

Will smoking marijuana do more harm than good?

What are the side effects of medical marijuana?

What form of cannabis is best to treat my symptoms with minimal impact on my mental state?

Acupuncture involves insertion and manipulation of needles at specific points in the body with the goal to relieve nausea, pain or other symptoms. Before acupuncture, check with your healthcare provider.

Aromatherapy

It is believed that mood and emotion can be altered by chemical messages sent to the brain by the aroma that comes from certain substances such as Roman chamomile, geranium, lavender and cedar wood. Most often cancer patients use aromatherapy to improve their quality of life.

Cannabis / marijuana

Cannabis is gaining a therapeutic role as an adjunct to cancer treatment. Increasing evidence supports the use of cannabis in the management of chemotherapy-induced nausea and for pain management as an addition or substitute for opioids.

Ask your physician if this is a good choice for you, and to help you find a registered provider who can prescribe medical marijuana. Remember to check on the legal aspects of using cannabis in your state.

Spiritual Support

MARY ANN

My magic was my belief in God, and somehow knowing that He wanted me to live through this.

Prayer, laying on of hands, and many forms of spiritual imagery or inner dialogue have helped patients find the higher strength within themselves to cope with cancer and other illness. Even those who have little or no connection with religion, often find themselves moved by the "spiritual emergency" of cancer.

ALTERNATIVE TREATMENTS

From time to time, a new product suddenly appears, and is promoted as a miraculous alternative to standard medical treatment. Most of the time, the claims are founded on a few poorly documented cases of alleged cures, and driven by nothing but the promoter's greed or ignorance.

It is easy to understand how a person undergoing treatment for a disease that is life threatening, may be tempted to pursue anything that promises a cure. Those who succumb to the temptation run the risk of disappointment, or medically disastrous results.

If you find yourself considering an unproven therapy, particularly if it is at the exclusion of a proven method, do yourself a favor: discuss your thoughts with your physician.

QUESTIONS TO ASK
YOUR DOCTOR:

What benefits can be expected from this therapy?

Do the known benefits outweigh the risks?

What side effects can be expected?

Will the therapy interfere with conventional treatment?

Will the therapy be covered by health insurance?

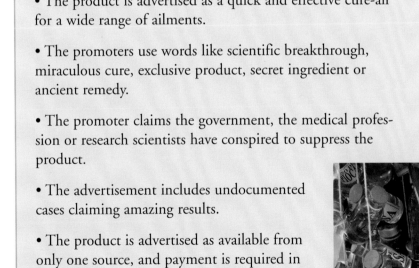

TIPS FOR SPOTTING FALSE CLAIMS

• The product is advertised as a quick and effective cure-all for a wide range of ailments.

• The promoters use words like scientific breakthrough, miraculous cure, exclusive product, secret ingredient or ancient remedy.

• The promoter claims the government, the medical profession or research scientists have conspired to suppress the product.

• The advertisement includes undocumented cases claiming amazing results.

• The product is advertised as available from only one source, and payment is required in advance.

• The promoter promises a "no-risk, money-back guarantee."

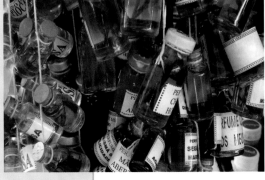

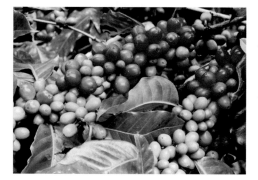

•••

As you go through your treatment, you'll realize that dealing with lung cancer requires that you leave no stone unturned, no tool unused. With the approval of your medical team, you may find that complementary therapies can play a valuable role in your treatment plan.

CHAPTER 10

CLINICAL TRIALS

WHAT ARE CLINICAL TRIALS?

Scientists are continually searching for better ways of dealing with cancer. This search is done in the form of clinical trials.

A clinical trial is an evaluation of a new way of managing cancer—with a new drug, a new procedure or a new diagnostic tool.

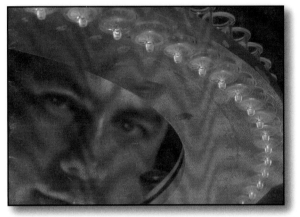

You may be reluctant to participate in what you might think is just an "experiment" with you as the "guinea pig". Nothing could be further from the truth. Clinical trials are conducted according to very specific guidelines developed by highly trained specialists, and carried out in steps, or phases.

Phase I trials assess the safety of the treatment in a small group of people.

Phase II trials assess the effectiveness. A larger group of patients are carefully monitored for improvement and for side effects.

Phase III trials are conducted on thousands of patients, in several medical centers across the country. To reach this stage the treatment method or drug must have demonstrated that it offers potential benefits, without unacceptable risks.

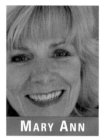

MARY ANN

My doctor asked me if I would join a trial he was running – a drug to make radiation more effective. I said, "Would you put your mother on it?" he said, "Absolutely." I told him to sign me up.

QUESTIONS TO ASK
YOUR DOCTOR:

- **Does being in a trial mean standard therapy has failed?**

- **Do you have other patients enrolled in trials?**

- **What trials are open in my area?**

HOW ARE CLINICAL TRIALS CONDUCTED?

The patients are selected for trials according to very specific criteria—age, stage of cancer, previous treatment, and so on, then divided into two groups by a random, computerized system. One group receives the new treatment, the other the best current treatment.

Every trial is conducted according to a protocol—a set of guidelines that spells out exactly what will be done and when. The trial is stopped if there are unacceptable side effects. The trial will also be stopped if it becomes obvious early on that either the new or the old treatment is definitely superior. In this case, all trial participants, both in the treatment and in the control groups, will be immediately switched to whichever treatment was found to be more effective.

In most cases, the trial runs the entire course—usually years, and the results are then compiled and analyzed. If the consensus among the researchers confirms the benefits, the drug or treatment will be made available to all patients. Many of today's "standard treatments" for cancer are based on methods that not so many years ago where considered "experimental" and were being studied in clinical trials.

Before the study is launched in a particular hospital, it is thoroughly reviewed by the hospital's Institutional Review Board, or IRB. An IRB is a committee of people, such as doctors, nurses, scientists, dentists, chaplains, social workers, attorneys and patients who are responsible for protecting clinical trial participants and making sure that the trials follow federal laws.

The IRB reviews and approves the protocol to make sure that it is based on reliable scientific evidence, and that there is good reason to believe that the treatment being evaluated will be significantly better. After a clinical trial begins, the IRB monitors the trial at least once a year and stops it if any safety concerns arise.

PARTICIPATING IN A CLINICAL TRIAL

If your physician does not mention trials, you may want to bring up the subject on your own. Generally, you or your physician can obtain information about ongoing trials from the National Cancer Institute's hotline called PDQ, or from the local chapter of the American Cancer Society.

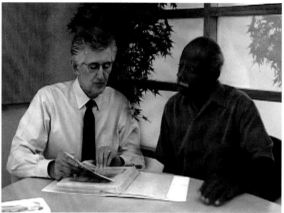

All trials have certain enrollment requirements. Some clinical trials only include patients who have not yet received treatment. Other trials test treatments for patients whose cancer has not gotten better.

You will also be evaluated regarding your performance status. Performance status is a term used to describe your overall health condition, based on the severity of your symptoms, your ability to care for yourself, and your general level of function. The purpose of the grading is to assign an objective measurement to your eligibility for a clinical trial.

If you qualify, and if you decide to proceed, you will be asked to sign an *informed consent form*, to show that you understand the issues involved, the expected benefits, the possible side effects, your rights and responsibilities, and the possible outcome.

You will be expected to follow the schedule of treatments and tests as closely as possible, in order to make the information obtained scientifically reliable.

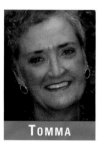

TOMMA

The good thing about trials is that your doctors follow you much more closely. You get life-long care, treatment, and follow up.

SANDRA: I had a physician friend of mine review the papers, and I also took them home, and had my husband review them too… I particularly liked that I would be carefully monitored. So I had no hesitation!

TOMMA

My doctor sat with my husband and me and spelled it all out. The goal for the trial, the risks... Wow, there was a lot of paperwork. All the stuff that can happen to you. I asked, "Should I be afraid of the trial?" And he said, "You should be more afraid of the tumor."

IS A TRIAL RIGHT FOR ME?

Some patients may be concerned about the safety of a trial. All reputable institutions conducting clinical trials feel that their most important responsibility is to protect patients through well-designed protocols, a dedicated Institutional Review Board (IRB) and a careful informed consent process.

For some patients, taking part in a clinical trial may be the best treatment choice. The benefits are many:

A clinical trial may allow you to gain access to new research developments before they are widely available to the public.

In addition, whether you are randomly assigned to the control group or to the treatment group, you will still enjoy a higher standard of care. That is because trial protocols usually call for more frequent tests, more frequent visits to the hospital, and more thorough examinations.

Last but not least, you will have the opportunity to help others by contributing to medical research.

QUESTIONS TO ASK
YOUR DOCTOR:

- **What is the purpose of the study?**

- **How long will the trial last?**

- **Will results of the trial be available to me?**

- **What is involved in terms of tests, treatments, and additional time commitments?**

- **What results can be reasonably expected in my particular case?**

What are some of the downsides to participating in clinical trials?

More than likely, you will be joining a Phase III trial, involving a drug or a method that has already been partially tested on smaller groups (Phase II), and will presumably be free of major side effects. Still, there may be unpleasant or even serious side effects to experimental treatment.

In addition, the clinical trial may require more of your time and attention than would a standard treatment, including trips to the study site, more treatment, hospital stays or complex dose requirements.

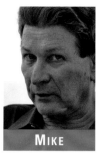

MIKE

When the doctor said, "research" I immediately thought I was going to be the lab rat. But then I looked into it, and it made sense. It was a no-lose situation. Eventually I felt very fortunate that I got to benefit from it.

HOW TO EVALUATE A CLINICAL TRIAL:

• How do I know the facility doing the study is reputable?

• What is involved in terms of tests, treatments, and additional time commitments?

• What results can be expected in my particular case?

• What are the currently accepted treatments and how do they compare to the trial?

• What would be my financial commitment?

• Will I need to be available for follow-up testing?

•••

Always remember that your participation is completely optional and voluntary. You can leave the trial at any time. If you drop out, you will not be penalized in any way, and you will still be entitled to the best standard treatment available.

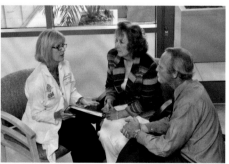

CHAPTER 11

LIFE AFTER CANCER

YOU, AGAIN...

As the treatments end and your energy and confidence return, you will learn how to move past the cancer experience. Gradually, less and less of your day will be occupied with trips to the hospital, and more of your time will be spent on your normal activities. You will find yourself moving from being a "patient" to being a "person" again.

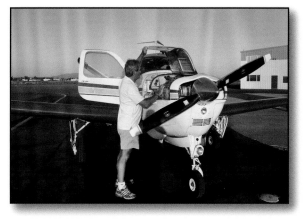

EMOTIONAL RECOVERY

A diagnosis of cancer impacts your self-esteem, your body image, even your outlook on survival. You probably realize that life will never be the same after such an experience. Seeing yourself differently and questioning your potential for survivorship may leave you with a sense of loss. Take time to grieve the loss. This grieving process is an important first step toward healing and moving forward.

Like many survivors, you may find that the cancer experience can be a powerful incentive to reorder your priorities; to eliminate from your life the unimportant negatives, and concentrate on enjoying the positives. You may decide to do something you always wanted to do—write poetry, travel, or spend more time with your grandchildren.

As you progress through treatment and recovery you may want to make an effort to find something enjoyable in every day, in every task. A bright moment that you can anticipate as a reward for your efforts, or a respite

QUESTIONS TO ASK
YOUR DOCTOR:

- **Is there any point in quitting smoking now?**
- **What factors are the greatest risks to my cancer recurring?**
- **What is the best cancer follow-up schedule for me?**
- **What should I recommend to my relatives about lung cancer screening?**
- **How can I get involved so I can help others afflicted by lung cancer?**

from your ordeals. You can celebrate your milestones, such as the first year anniversary of being cancer-free, or a negative PET/CT report.

One of the most challenging, but also most rewarding lifestyle changes is stress reduction. Easier said than done at a time when you have to deal with a life threatening illness, financial challenges, decreased ability to work, and strained personal relationships.

The first step in reducing stress in your life is to identify the stressors. Make a list of the main items that provoke anxiety. Then think creatively how you can eliminate them, one by one.

Indecision about treatment choices? Have an in-depth discussion with your healthcare team, and plan a course of action.

Financial worries? Consult your accountant, someone who is helping you with your health plan, or a representative from the hospital business office. If necessary, consider a loan from a bank or from a relative.

Anxiety about survival? Get help from a counselor who is trained in dealing with cancer-related issues. Distract yourself with a new hobby, join a new social group or take a community class.

Complementary therapies such as relaxation, exercises, yoga, or meditation, described in an earlier chapter, can accomplish wonders in stress management, and may even help you in your personal and professional life as well.

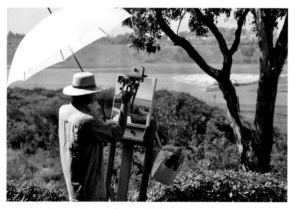

A creative endeavor helps reduce stress.

HEALTHY HABITS

This may be a good time to adopt healthy habits.

No, it is not too late to stop smoking. There is compelling evidence that patients who continue smoking reduce the effectiveness of their treatment, and increase the chances of developing another cancer.

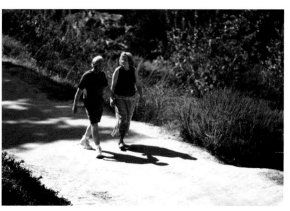

In addition, stopping smoking will improve your body's ability to cope with the side effects of treatment. You will heal faster and tolerate chemotherapy and radiation better.

Exercise brings a variety of health benefits.

Physical activity will help you stay stronger and fight any fatigue that still may be lingering. There is also evidence that moderate physical exercise can improve the work of the immune system, and help protect you against cancer and other diseases.

If your lung capacity has been compromised by surgery or by treatment, you may need to learn new breathing techniques that make better use of both your chest and abdominal muscles. Pulmonary rehabilitation can work wonders to increase your breathing capacity. There is no such thing as getting too much oxygen into your system.

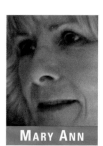

MARY ANN

Good Nutrition

Good nutrition may speed your healing after surgery. A balanced diet, with proper amounts of protein, fats, carbohydrates, and a multi-vitamin supplement will help you feel younger and stay healthier.

Exercise was my best drug. It helped me physically, it helped me mentally, it helped me emotionally. The spinning makes your lungs open up and breath, and the endorphins calm you down. There is nothing better!

If weight loss is a problem, consider supplementing your diet with Carnation Instant Breakfast made with whole milk or added to a milk shake. Ensure and Boost are also good supplements for protein and calories. These can be added to milkshakes as well. Your physician may recommend a medication to stimulate your appetite.

REGULAR FOLLOW-UP

Even after the most complete treatment, there's always a chance that cancer will recur. Regular follow-up is vital. The National Comprehensive Cancer Network (NCCN), an alliance of the world's leading cancer centers, has developed guidelines for a follow-up schedule. Whether it is your surgeon, oncologist or primary physician, it's important to have a single person in charge, to ensure continuity of care.

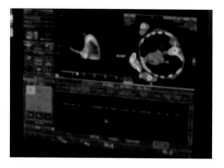

If you have no symptoms, and there is good reason to expect that you are cured, you may be seen every three months for the first two years. After that you will be seen twice a year for three years, and once a year thereafter.

Tests may include PET or CT scans to determine if there is any evidence of cancer return. Often the tests will focus on specific symptoms that you may have, rather than be a random search for recurrence.

ADVICE FOR OTHERS

Screening and early detection for lung cancer is gradually improving. A large clinical trial called the National Lung Screening Trial (NLST) found that computed tomography (CT) scans detect lung cancer at an earlier, more curable stage compared to traditional X-rays resulting in 20% fewer deaths.

Another approach uses newer, more sensitive tests to look for cancer cells in sputum samples.

Current studies are looking at new tests to determine whether they are useful in finding lung cancers at an earlier stage. You may want to encourage your smoking friends to seek their physicians' advice about getting screened.

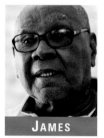

ALI

Cancer made me less tolerant of people who complain about issues that are really insignificant. What the hell do these people have to complain about? "You broke your nail? Lost the golf game? BMW need repairs? How dreadful! Try living with cancer."

JAMES

I walk two to four miles every day. If you can't walk two miles, walk one. Walk 100 yards. All you can manage is eight steps across your room? OK. Tomorrow try nine steps.

POST-TREATMENT DEPRESSION

Chemotherapy is over. Radiation therapy ended. The surgical scars are healed. And yet that is when you suddenly experience a big let down, and become depressed.

This is a common occurrence among cancer patients. When treatments end, you may not only feel abandoned by your doctors, but also vulnerable since you are not actively fighting the disease. You may find that the continual threat of recurrence never goes away and that the anxiety inhibits you from leading a fulfilling life.

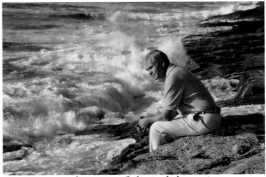

Learn the signs of clinical depression.

If this anxiety interferes with your quality of life or ability to function, ask your physician for a referral to a counselor. You may also consider joining a support group consisting of other recent "treatment graduates".

In this group you may share with others who are just beginning treatment that they will make it through. Giving back to others with lung cancer may give you a real sense of purpose. If you are physically able, you may want to volunteer at the cancer center or the hospital where you received your treatment.

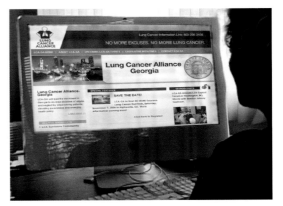

Survivors can become cancer advocates.

Another way to contribute to the cause is to become an advocate for a cure for lung cancer. This can be done while sitting at a computer. You can network with others and write letters to people of influence regarding research and treatment for lung cancer. The sky's the limit! You are a survivor and have a wealth of understanding and experience to share with others.

MARY ANN: How can something good come out of an experience like cancer? Well, you get a better perspective on things. You learn not to sweat the little stuff. And it helped me learn to give of myself. And there is no greater satisfaction than knowing you have helped another human being.

•••

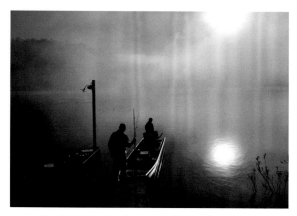

Looking forward to many beautiful dawns...

Ultimately, there is no substitute for the healing effect of time. With each passing week, you will adjust better and better to the new order of priorities and issues. As you complete your treatments, cancer may move gradually from your present into your past, to be replaced with anticipation of a brighter future.

CHAPTER 12

ADVANCED CANCER

FACING THE FUTURE

Writing chapters about cancer treatment is an easy task. Surgical techniques or chemotherapy regimens are fairly standard, and the information I presented very likely applies to your case. But giving you advice on how to face the prospect of dying if your treatments fail is a daunting task.

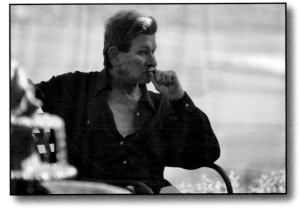

Different people deal with end-of-life issues in different ways. Some accept the prognosis and concentrate on preparing for the inevitable. Others choose to fight the disease till the very end. Most will go through both of these phases at some point in their treatment.

The best – in fact, the only – advice I can give you is to do what feels right. As you talk to your medical team, to other survivors, and to your loved ones, you will know what is best for you. You will know whether it is your time to sit down and get your affairs in order, or to muster up the strength for one more round of chemo.

No written chapter can be a substitute to an in-depth discussion with a loved one or with your own healthcare provider.

Much of the information that follows is somewhat generic. Take from it what applies to you. You may find that the most valuable portion of this chapter is what other survivors say. The thoughts of those who have been down this path before you.

QUESTIONS TO ASK
YOUR DOCTOR:

- **What treatment options are available to me at this stage?**

- **Are there other specialists I should consult?**

- **Tell me about palliative care.**

- **Tell me about the hospice experience.**

IF TREATMENT FAILS

If you were diagnosed with an advanced stage of lung cancer, you started your treatments knowing that your life expectancy might be limited. What no one can tell you is whether you will be among those who survive, or among those whose treatments fail. How and when will you know?

At some point, you may become aware of changes in your body and your ability to function. You may find yourself feeling more tired. You may need more help with completing daily activities such as bathing, dressing, and eating. Your hospitalizations become longer and more frequent. Your chemotherapy or radiation therapy is no longer effective. Your time between blood transfusions becomes shorter and shorter. Your physicians seem less willing to recommend additional treatments.

You might ask yourself, what does this mean? Am I too tired or too demoralized to go on? Is my healthcare team giving up? What is the right thing to do?

Such questions and worries are normal reactions when you begin to realize that your chance of survival is poor and that the cancer treatments are failing.

QUALITY VS. QUANTITY

How will you know when it is time to accept the fact that you are dying? This realization may come to you when you decide that the discomfort of a bronchoscopy to relieve yet another bronchial obstruction is not worth the short-lived relief. Or that the new round of chemo takes away more energy than it gives you. Or that the pain medications rob you of your ability to enjoy the loved ones around you. In other words, the price in pain and discomfort per day of life is too high.

As you consider these issues, the insight will come to you, and you will know what the right thing to do is.

This is the point at which you may want to begin striving for more quality, instead of quantity, in your life. In other words, your focus might gradually change from extending the number of days or weeks that you live, to improving the quality of the last portion of your life. You may choose two weeks filled with things you enjoy doing, over four weeks of incapacitating side effects.

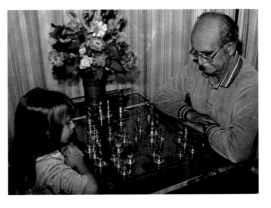

PLANNING FOR THE END OF LIFE

Plan for the last stages of your life the same way you planned for the first stages of your treatment.

The earlier you discuss your concerns with your medical team, the greater control you will retain. If no one on your team is experienced with end-of-life management, ask to be referred to a specialist.

END-OF-LIFE DECISIONS

- Managing symptoms, such as shortness of breath or pain
- Deciding what drugs or treatments you wish to have
- Getting the most out of your interaction with your loved ones
- Ordering your financial affairs and commitments

QUESTIONS TO ASK
YOUR DOCTOR:

- **Do I really need powerful drugs to control my pain?**

- **Is it OK if I take as little pain medication as possible?**

- **How long can I take narcotics for pain without getting addicted?**

PALLIATIVE CARE

We don't yet have the technology to cure all lung cancers, but we have made enormous progress in understanding how we can make the quality of life better for patients. Do take advantage of everything that is available to you. There might be more than you can imagine.

Reducing symptoms and improving life quality is sometimes referred to as *palliative care.* The goal of palliative care is not to cure your cancer, but to make you more comfortable.

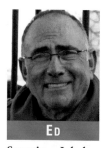

ED

Sometimes I do have to talk about dying. Some people don't like to hear that. Well, I tell them to get lost. Don't feel like you have to apologize for having to die.

One of the fears that many patients report is dealing with symptoms such as pain or shortness of breath. Do not accept these symptoms as inevitable. There are excellent drugs available today to help relieve or eliminate your pain, and yet leave you alert enough to interact with those around you. There are also interventions that help treat shortness of breath. Many cancer centers have a palliative care team who will work with you to provide symptom management, pain control and comfort measures.

Ask your physicians which interventions are most likely to be effective in your case. Accepting the fact that you will not be cured doesn't mean you need to accept any pain or discomfort.

HOSPICE CARE

Many patients and family members are uncomfortable with the term "hospice." They may feel that they will not be cared for properly or that feeding will be withdrawn. This could not be further from the truth. Hospice actually has many benefits that support not just the patient but the entire family. Hospice is a specialized form of care for patients who are at an advanced stage of their terminal illness. Hospice programs are designed to keep a patient close to family and friends whenever possible. Although many hospice programs are centered in the home, patients in nursing homes or assisted living facilities can receive hospice care as well.

A complete hospice team includes physicians, nurses, nutritionists, physical therapists, social workers, spiritual care advisors and any other specialists needed to maintain your comfort for as long as possible. Many hospice programs will also focus on the well being of your loved ones.

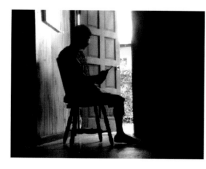

Typically, in a hospice experience, a comfortable hospital-style bed will be brought to your home. Your loved ones will administer as much of the daily care as you and they are comfortable with. The rest of the care will be delivered by various members of the hospice team when they come to see you in your home at pre-appointed times.

Hospice is available for patients of any age, religion, race, and illness. It provides support to the patient and to family or caregivers. Hospice care is covered under Medicare, Medical/Medicaid, most private insurances, HMOs and other managed care organizations.

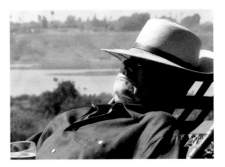

In a way, hospice care combines the best of both worlds: you will be in your own familiar home surroundings, and yet your medical professionals will be available 24-7, just as in a hospital setting.

ADVANCE CARE PLANNING

A time will come when you will no longer feel confident in deciding how to manage the financial and other tasks in your life, or how to communicate your wishes. This is when your advance care planning will prove to be most useful.

What is advance care planning? *Advance care planning* is a process where an individual talks with others about his or her wishes with regard to future healthcare, legal, and financial matters. Included in this discussion are the patient's wishes about end-of-life care and decisions about life prolonging medical treatments. Do you want to have CPR if your breathing or heart stops? Do you want to be put on a respirator or breathing machine if you are unable to breathe on your own? Do you want artificial tube feedings? These are examples of prolonged medical treatments about which you can make decisions in advance.

What is the next step? After discussing your choices and wishes with family, significant others, and healthcare providers, it is important to have them documented and distributed to those involved in your care.

Decisions regarding healthcare are documented on a form called Advance Healthcare Directive.

Since some contingencies cannot be anticipated in a written document, no matter how detailed, you may also want to grant the Durable Power of Attorney for Healthcare or Medical Power of Attorney to a trusted person.

QUESTIONS TO ASK
YOUR DOCTOR:

• **Who can help me draw up documents such as advance directives, etc?**

• **Are there support groups my loved ones can join?**

• **How do I decide if it is time to stop treatment?**

• **What can I do to prepare for my death?**

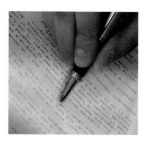

This person will then be empowered to make decisions on your behalf when you are no longer able to do so.

It is not necessary to have an attorney to create an Advance Healthcare Directive. You can find the forms on the internet, or at your local hospital.

Advance Healthcare Directives cannot be used for financial affairs or estate planning. For these, you should consult an attorney for information about documents dealing with living trusts, last wills and testaments, assets, and Financial Durable Powers of Attorney.

An individual has the right to revoke their Advance Healthcare Directives, and to change their wishes regarding financial affairs. Therefore, it is important to review these documents periodically to reflect your current wishes.

Don't think of preparing your advance directives as an indication of giving up the battle. A well conceived and documented plan will allow you and your loved ones to concentrate on quality time with you, instead of on last minute paperwork.

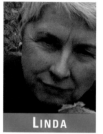

LINDA

I know doctors have to be honest, but they also need to give patients more hope. There is always time to take hope away. It serves no purpose to say, "There is nothing we can do."

ED: Look, they counted 43 tumors in me when I was diagnosed, and they gave me six months. That was eleven years ago. You have to keep fighting. Till they close the lid.

Most of us who are terminal do come to grips with the inevitable. I will probably die from lung cancer. But look, how wonderful if you can get an extra five years, or one year. Just say, I can win.

ED - 15 years after diagnosis: Still feel the same way.

HELPING YOUR LOVED ONES

When you were first diagnosed with lung cancer, it was probably difficult for your loved ones to figure out how to relate to you. When you and they realize that you are going to die from this disease, it's even more difficult for them to interact with you. For most people, it is new, confusing territory.

Perhaps the best course for you to take, as you probably did in the beginning, is to be the first one to bring up the issue. Say what is on your mind. Share your thoughts, your fears, and your hopes.

Friends who come visit you may be equally at a loss for what to say. You may need to be the one to get the conversation going. It might be something like, "I know I look like hell... I realize this is a shock to you... I know that it's difficult to think of something to say but it's so nice of you to come and feel free to just sit with me a bit... It's hard to talk and breathe, so I'll just listen. Tell me about your day..."

ED

I put all my old home movies and slides on DVD. Costco does it. And I am going to title and label everything. To help them remember the good times. To leave a footprint.

LEAVING A LEGACY

You probably want your family and loved ones to remember you not by how you looked in your last days, but by the important things you have done, or by happier moments you have shared with them.

Your legacy does not need to be an important invention, or a set of novels you have written, or a house you have built. You may not realize it right now, but decades after you are gone, your family will cherish things that may seem completely unimportant to you now.

Why not pull out old albums and take the time to label the photos so that those who come after you will remember the occasions? Or how about organizing your favorite recipes, and adding a few personal suggestions to them? Have you considered writing—or better yet, recording—messages for your grandchildren? The possibilities are endless. Not only will the work result in something tangible that will probably survive in your family for generations, but it will also provide you with a wonderful opportunity to do something fun with your loved ones.

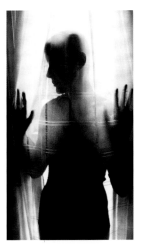

Survivor Lou plans to produce a one-woman show about her experience.

•••

You, your loved ones, and your medical team may realize that you have entered the last stages of your life. There will be days when there is fear and despair and anger and weakness, and there will be days with strength and acceptance and understanding.

ED: I do have down days. Days when you feel, "Enough already. I just want to pack it in." What helps? My walking. I walk two to four miles every day. Rain or shine. Every single day. I think. I talk to my dead dad. I get centered. Then I go to the Y and do water aerobics with the blue haired ladies...

Stay alive, stay positive. We know in advance it's "game over." But it must be on our terms. I ask, Where is it written when Ed is going to die? I'll die when I am good and ready, by golly. I am not into being underground in a cheap pine box.

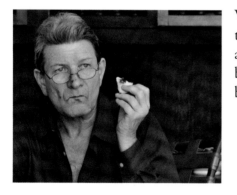

What no one knows is when your life will actually end. Until then, make the most of your time – enjoy your loved ones and your environment. And, above all, take the time to look back, and relish all the things you have done right, and all the battles you have won.

CHAPTER 13

A GUIDE FOR YOUR PARTNER

"FOR BETTER OR FOR WORSE..."

If you are the spouse or life partner of someone who has just been diagnosed with lung cancer, now is the time to remember: you made a commitment to be there, during good times and bad times. Your spouse needs you now probably more than ever.

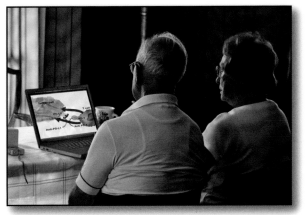

Even if yours is not a long-term relationship—perhaps you just met, or you are the patient's closest or only friend—you should realize that you now have an opportunity to do something truly meaningful, something that will make a real difference in another human being's life. Consider this opportunity a gift not to be refused.

A NOTE ON MY WORDING

To avoid long lists of possible relationships, I'll be using "partner" or "spouse" to mean you, the caregiver, whatever your special relationship may be—husband, wife, sister, best friend, life partner... I'll also use he, she, her or him randomly and interchangeably to avoid the clumsy "s/he" or "him/her" neo-pronouns.

WHAT IS LUNG CANCER?

You have probably heard that lung cancer is not a good disease. Don't leap to generalizations. A lot depends on how early the lung cancer is diagnosed. Very often, when the lung cancer was found as a tiny tumor, usually on a routine study, in a patient who had no symptoms, treatment can be very effective, and cure is often possible.

Begin by reviewing the appropriate chapters of this book with your partner. Understanding the disease will help you regain a feeling of control over your life.

UNDERSTANDING YOUR FEELINGS

"I have lung cancer" may be the most painful words you'll ever hear from someone you love. Words that cause shock, disbelief, and confusion, and make you wonder, "Is my loved one going to die?"

Finding yourself responsible for emotional and physical support is challenging. You're probably in as much pain and turmoil as your partner, but your burden may be heavier. Not only do you have to provide the support to your loved one, but you also have to deal with your own feelings.

You may feel overwhelmed by the sense that somehow you must make it all better, and be frustrated when you find out you can't. There is no easy answer, and no shortcut. You are facing a serious problem, and it is normal to feel scared, confused, and weak. Acknowledge these feelings. You can be strong and supportive without holding everything inside. In fact, sharing your feelings honestly is the best thing you can do to strengthen the relationship.

If you find it too hard to express these feelings to your partner, you can find a support person for yourself. A friend, another family member, a religious leader, a counselor, or a support group can help you verbalize what you are feeling, sort it all out, and work on a plan of action.

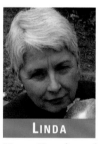

LINDA

Hope. You always have to have hope. You have to stand up and fight. You can't give up. As long as Ed keeps fighting, I'll keep fighting for him.

The first weeks after the diagnosis may feel like an emotional roller coaster. The swings of feelings are painful and exhausting, but they are normal. With time the emotional tidal waves fade to be mere ripples in a pool, and you find that you can deal with them.

What Do I Do Now?

One of the most constructive actions you can take is to get involved in your spouse's care. Read the general chapters in this book, then concentrate on the chapters that discuss the specific type of treatment that he will have. Learn all you can about the disease and the most current treatment options.

Accompany your spouse on visits to the healthcare specialists. Your presence will provide emotional support and a second set of ears.

Bring a list of questions you want answered. Take notes, or use a voice recorder. If at first you are confused, don't worry. Lung cancer treatment is a complex topic, and no one can grasp all the details on the first pass.

If either of you feel you need a second opinion, don't hesitate to ask for a referral, or seek one on your own. For something as important as cancer treatment, you should leave no avenue unexplored, and no reputable physician will resent your request.

A diagnosis of cancer is seldom an emergency. You and your partner have several weeks to make important treatment decisions. Don't let anyone rush you.

Above all, remember that it is the patient who makes the final decisions about treatment choices. Being supportive and helpful does not mean taking over completely.

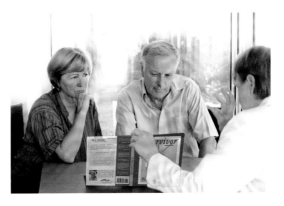

Questions to Ask Your Doctor:

- Do you have any pamphlets, videos, or DVD's about lung cancer that we can take home and review?

- Who would you recommend we see for a second opinion?

- Can you put us in touch with others who you treated for this type of cancer, and with their partners?

- Will chemotherapy cause hair to fall out?

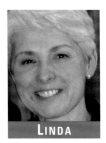

LINDA

If something happens to Ed... I'll be devastated, but I'll know that I have done everything possible to keep him alive as long as possible.

WHAT YOUR SPOUSE NEEDS FROM YOU

Emotional Support

Emotional support is perhaps the single most important thing you can contribute. Knowing that you will be there, no matter what, will help your spouse deal with the diagnosis, and tolerate the treatments.

If you find verbal communication to be difficult, and choose to hide in your job or in an outside activity, your spouse may perceive this behavior as a withdrawal of your love. Her well-being depends on your willingness to communicate openly. You don't need to make long speeches. Holding hands, sitting close, putting an arm around her, will communicate how much she means to you in ways words can't express.

Most people are upset by tearful outbursts. But tears are a healthy response. Both of you know that there is no easy fix, and to pretend otherwise only delays the grieving that must take place before healing begins.

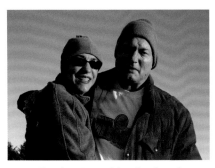

Stephanie and her husband

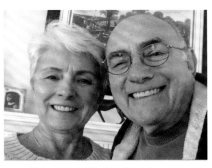

Ed with wife Linda 15 years

STEPHANIE: When I was diagnosed with the lung and the breast cancers, my husband was dying of bladder cancer. All I could think off was that my eight year old daughter would wind up an orphan. He was amazing! He was on chemo, yet he somehow rallied enough to take care of me for eight months. And as soon as I was able to go to work, he let himself go. And died a couple of weeks later. He was my rock!

LINDA - 15 years after diagnosis: As long as Ed is willing to fight, I'll fight right alongside him.

SIMPLE TECHNIQUES TO IMPROVE COMMUNICATIONS:

• Make opening statements that let your partner know you're willing to listen. Comments like, "How do you feel about...," let her know it's okay to open up on an emotional level.

• Reassure her that she has been truly understood by repeating what you heard in your own words: "So you are saying that..."

• Use nonverbal, body language, techniques to communicate. Hand holding, and looking at her when she speaks, tell her that your love and concern are real.

• Avoid judgmental comments like, "You shouldn't...," or, "Don't say that." Such statements block true communication by minimizing or invalidating the other person's feelings.

• Be careful with comments like, "Don't worry," or, "Nothing will happen." Having a positive attitude doesn't mean being unrealistic.

• Be sensitive to the moment. If your loved one is in a positive state of mind and wants to discuss vacation plans, don't sour the mood by turning the conversation to chemotherapy.

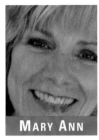

MARY ANN

My husband was by my side at every step. Some nights we hugged and cried together. Other nights we went out and had fun. When my hair started shedding, and I shaved my head, he said I looked beautiful. That meant the world to me.

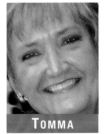

TOMMA

My husband is a glass half empty kind of guy. He was willing to do anything to help me, but he was still sure he would be planning my funeral. So I had to help him. He has grown a lot from this experience.

Anger is also a normal response that needs an outlet. The patient may lash out at the closest person during such times. Despite what he says, he is not angry at you, but at his loss of control over his life. This stage will pass faster if you help direct that anger into action against the cancer.

Some patients withdraw and refuse to share their feelings, rejecting your efforts at being close. This may be the most difficult reaction to deal with, and may require outside help to reestablish open communications.

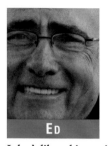

ED

I don't like taking pain pills. I want to know where I am at. So sometimes I am in pain. And my wife hates it, and she yells at me. And it upsets me. But what I need to remember is that she too needs help. Because she is going through living hell.

There is scientific evidence that a positive mind-set can lead to an improved outcome. A supportive and upbeat attitude on your part will be contagious and is one of the best ways to help him through the weeks or months of treatment.

Sexual Intimacy

When is the right time for resuming sexual relations? There is nothing about cancer or its treatment that would prevent intimate contact. The deciding factor is your partner's, and your, readiness.

Preoccupation with the cancer and its treatment may wipe out any interest in sexual intimacy. There are small things you can do to rekindle this interest. Make a date, offer a foot rub, take a shower together, watch a romantic movie. Try new positions that may be more comfortable.

Help with Daily Activities

Surgery, chemotherapy, and emotional stress may lead to physical exhaustion, and your spouse may look like she needs your help even with the simplest daily activities. The difficult part may be determining how much help she really wants. Too much help may be as inappropriate as too little. The simple solution: just ask!

SUGGESTIONS FOR FRIENDS WHO WANT TO HELP

- Stop by and bring a newspaper.

- Bring the mail or other materials from the office.

- Help redecorate a room.

- Organize a getaway weekend for both of you.

- Drop by and watch a favorite TV program.

- Drive to a chemotherapy session.

- Invite the whole family out for a meal.

In the early stages of treatment the patient is often overcome with an excess of well-wishing friends and relatives. Your job may be to act as the gatekeeper, and delegate specific tasks to various people so everyone feels involved.

Financial or Insurance Issues

You also may be required to deal with financial or insurance issues. Be meticulous. A minor mistake in bookkeeping on your part may have serious financial consequences.

DEALING WITH INSURANCE:
HOW TO MAKE AN UNPLESANT TASK EASIER

• Contact your insurance company at the time of diagnosis to find out their policies on hospital admissions, additional medical opinions, filing of claims and billing, etc.

• Keep a written record of your contacts with insurance company representatives, including names, dates, and times.

• Write down appointment dates and doctors' names. Get a copy of all billing forms, which should include procedures, medications, and supplies used.

• Keep all bills, charges, and related forms together in one place for easy retrieval later.

• Don't forget to keep up insurance premiums. You'll be glad you remembered this critical step later.

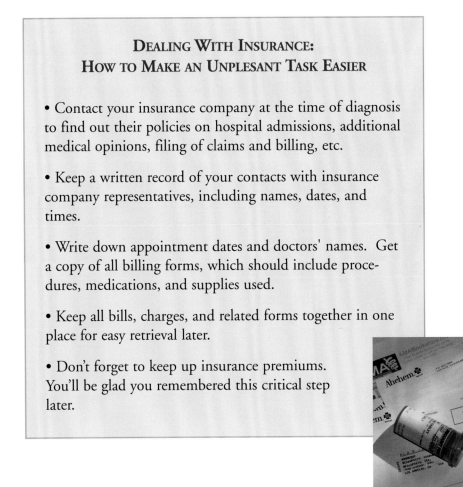

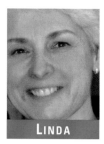

LINDA

I am a pretty laid back person. But when it comes to keeping my husband alive, I'll stand up to anybody!

MEETING YOUR OWN NEEDS

Finding Support For You

The combination of emotional stress, your regular work, and added activities around the home can take a toll on you. If you start to feel overwhelmed, make a list of tasks that need to be done on a daily basis (food preparation, house cleaning, etc). Try to concentrate on activities that really are essential, and put off the unnecessary niceties. Then seek assistance from family or friends whenever you need. A simple request may be all they are waiting for to pitch in.

Fear, anxiety and stress can tire you even more than physical work. Find a close friend or family member who can help ease the emotional burden you carry. Don't be afraid to let your pride down and share how you feel.

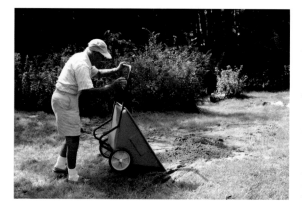

Talking to other partners of lung cancer patients and participating in support groups will also help you figure out how to cope.

And sometimes just a "boys" or "girls" night out might work wonders for your mood, and your energy.

Remember, you can't afford to exhaust yourself physically or emotionally.

● ● ●

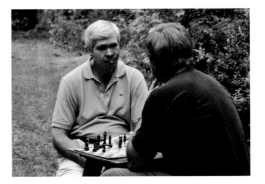

Going through the lung cancer experience with your partner may be one of the most trying transitions in your life.   Do your best. You may find that it leads to discovering new friendships, and strenghtening the bonds with your loved ones.

GLOSSARY

Adjuvant therapy
A treatment that is used in addition (as an adjunct) to the main treatment. For example, chemotherapy after surgery.

Advance directives
Legal documents that describe your wishes in future medical situations in case you are unable to make your own decisions.

Alternative therapy
A treatment that is considered unconventional and has no scientifically proven benefit.

Alveoli
Airsacs at the end of bronchial passages in the lungs.

Antiemetics
Drugs that prevent nausea and vomiting.

Antioxidants
Compounds that protect the body against damage by molecules known as free radicals.

Benign
Not cancerous.

Biopsy
Removal of tissues or cells from the body for microscopic examination.

Brachytherapy
Radiation therapy delivered by implanting radioactive seeds.

Bronchoscope
A flexible tube equipped with a light, video camera and biopsy tool that is inserted through the breathing passages to obtain images or tissue samples of lung tissue.

Cannabis / marijuana
A compound, illegal in some states, that may be effective in controlling some cancer symptoms, such as pain or nausea.

Carcinoma in situ
The earliest stage of cancer in which the tumor is confined to the most superficial site where it started.

Chemotherapy
A cancer treatment that uses specific drugs, either intravenously or orally, to destroy cancerous cells.

Chest tube
Flexible tube inserted into the chest cavity and attached to a suction device to remove air, blood or fluid and to keep the lung inflated.

Clinical trials
Studies that compare a standard treatment with a newly developed treatment.

Combination chemotherapy
The use of two or more drugs to treat cancer.

Complementary therapy
Therapies that are used in addition to standard treatments. Often effective in relieving side effects of treatment, reducing stress, and enhancing well-being.

Computerized tomography
(CT or CAT scan)
An imaging procedure that combines X-rays with a computer to produce detailed pictures of the organs.

Cyberknife
A device used to deliver radiation therapy with more precision. It is not a surgical tool.

EBUS
Endobronchial ultrasound – a tool used to help evaluate the extent of the tumor within the lungs. Also called EUS.

External beam radiation
Radiation delivered by a source (linear accelerator) outside the body.

Gene
A segment of genetic material (DNA) that carries hereditary information.

Genomic testing
Analysis of the genetic composition of the tumor with the goal of finding the most suitable therapy.

Hospice
End-of-life care that provides support while keeping the patient as close to the home environment as possible.

Intravenous (IV)
Delivered into a vein.

Immunotherapy
Also called targeted therapy.

Lobectomy
Surgical removal of a lobe of the lung.

Lymph nodes
Small bean-shaped organs that filter out germs and abnormal cells. They are connected by lymph ducts.

Magnetic resonance imaging (MRI)
An imaging method that combines magnetic fields, radio waves, and a computer to produce detailed pictures of the inside of the body.

Malignant
Cancerous.

Margin
The edge of removed tissue. A negative, or clear, margin has no cancer cells. A positive margin means that cancer cells were found at the edge of the tissue removed.

Marijuana
See cannabis.

Mediastinum
The area behind the breast bone, between the lungs, containing the trachea, heart, major blood vessels and lymph nodes.

Metastasis
The spread of cancer cells from the primary (original) site to other sites in the body.

Neoadjuvant therapy
Treatment, such as chemotherapy, that is administered prior to the primary treatment, such as surgery.

Palliative therapy
Treatment to help patients live more comfortably, rather than to cure them.

Personalised medicine
A treatment plan tailored to a specific patient's condition.

Pleura
Membrane lining the chest wall and the lungs, forming the pleural cavity.

Pneumothorax
Collapse of the lung due to air leakage into the pleural cavity.

Prognosis
A prediction of the likely outcome of a disease, or chance of survival, in a particular patient.

Proton therapy
A treatment that uses beams of protons, instead of photons, like radiation therapy does.

Radiation oncology
A specialty that uses various forms of radiation to treat cancer.

Radiation therapy
A treatment that uses high doses of radiation to treat or control cancer.

Recurrence
Cancer return after treatment. Local recurrence means that it has returned to the original site. Regional recurrence means that it has returned to tissues near the original site. Distant recurrence means that it has spread to other organs.

Resection
Surgery that removes part of, or all of, an organ.

SBRT
Stereotactic Body Radiation Therapy.

SRS
Stereotactic radiosurgery is a non-surgical radiation therapy used to treat small tumors.

Stage
A classification of the extent of the cancer.

Surgical oncology
A surgical subspecialty that focuses on treating cancer surgically.

Targeted therapy
Therapy designed to attack cancer cells specifically.

Thoracotomy
Incision in the chest wall to access the lungs during surgery.

TNM system
A staging system for cancer based on three key pieces of information: T, size of tumor, N, cancer spread to nearby nodes, and M cancer metastasis to other organs.

Tumor
An abnormal growth of cells that can be benign or malignant.

Ultrasound
A painless, noninvasive imaging method that uses high-frequency sound waves to locate and measure tumors and other abnormal growths in the body.

QUESTIONS TO ASK
YOUR HEALTHCARE PROVIDERS

This section contains questions gathered from the book. They are broken down by chapters with space for your own notes. Feel free to tear out or cut out these pages, and use them as reminders of what you want to discuss.

CHAPTER 1: FACING LUNG CANCER

QUESTIONS TO ASK YOUR DOCTOR:

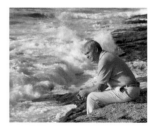

• How do other people deal with this diagnosis?

• How do I get rid of the guilt I feel about smoking?

• How can I help my loved ones handle their feelings about my diagnosis?

• Can I bring members of my family, or a friend, to talk to you directly?

• What should I tell my loved ones about my condition?

• Can you refer me to a counselor or to a support group specializing in lung cancer?

• Is there a multidisciplinary lung cancer team in the facility where you practice?

• Could you give me the names of specialists you think I should see?

• How about another set of names so I can choose the specialist(s) I like best?

• Tell me about your, or your colleagues' experience in dealing with lung cancer.

• Could you forward my chart, test results, and my biopsy slides to the doctor who is going to give me a second opinion?

• Can you give me the name of a lung cancer expert who can give me a second opinion?

CHAPTER 3: STAGING

QUESTIONS TO ASK YOUR DOCTOR:

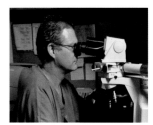

• What type of cancer do I have?

• What is the size of the tumor?

• What kind of tests will help determine if the cancer has spread?

NOTES

CHAPTER 4: TREATMENT OPTIONS

QUESTIONS TO ASK YOUR DOCTOR:

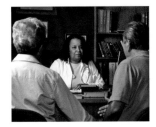

• What is the goal of my treatment – attempt to cure, or manage symptoms and improve quality of life?

• Why are we starting with surgery, and then giving me chemotherapy? My friend had the opposite.

• Do you have a team of doctors working with you on my case? If not, why not?

NOTES

CHAPTER 5: SURGERY

QUESTIONS TO ASK YOUR ANESTHESIOLOGIST:

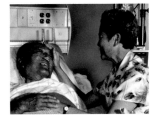

• Will you give me something to help me relax before the procedure?

• How long will it take me to get back to normal after the sedation? What are the side effects of sedation?

• If I have general anesthesia, how long will it take me to get back to normal?

• Will you give me something to control the pain after I wake up from the anesthetic?

QUESTIONS TO ASK YOUR SURGEON:

• What type of procedure do you think is best for me?

• What is the latest information about this type of cancer surgery?

• Could I meet with some of the patients who had this procedure before?

• How much pain should I expect after the procedure?

• How long before I can go back to my regular work or leisure activities?

• Will there be any long term effects?

• What follow-up visits do you recommend?

• How much lung will be removed?

• How will the removal of lung tissue affect my breathing?

• How much pain should I expect in the first few days after the procedure?

• How long can I take narcotics for pain without getting addicted?

• Do I need to arrange to have someone to help me with daily activities?

• How long before I can go back to my regular work or leisure activities?

CHAPTER 6: RADIATION THERAPY

QUESTIONS TO ASK YOUR DOCTOR:

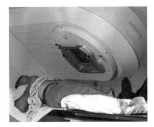

• Why do I need radiation therapy?

• How will I evaluate the effectiveness of the treatments?

• Can I continue my usual work or exercise schedule?

• Can I miss a few treatments?

• Can I arrange to be treated elsewhere if I am traveling?

• What side effects, if they occur, should I report immediately?

NOTES

CHAPTER 7: CHEMOTHERAPY

QUESTIONS TO ASK YOUR DOCTOR:

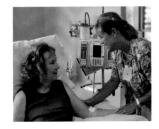

• Do I need chemotherapy? Why?

• What drugs do you recommend?

• What are the benefits and risks of chemotherapy?

• How successful is this treatment for the type of cancer I have?

• How will you evaluate the effectiveness of the treatments?

• What side effects will I experience?

• Can I work while I'm having chemotherapy?

• Can I travel between treatments (short business or pleasure trips)?

• What other limitations can I expect?

• How can I manage nausea?

• Will I be given medications to treat side effects?

• Can I take public transportation home after treatments?

• Can I take vitamins or herbs if I choose?

• Will my chemo be given IV or in pill form?

• How will I know if the pills are working?

• What side effects can I expect?

Chapter 8: Targeted Therapy and Immunotherapy

Questions to Ask Your Doctor:

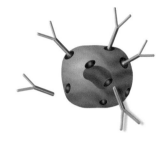

• Can my tumor be treated with targeted therapy? If not, why not?

• What drugs do you recommend?

• What side effects can I expect with this treatment?

• Will I be given medications to treat side effects?

• What are the benefits and risks of targeted therapy?

• How successful is this treatment for the type of cancer I have?

• How will you evaluate the effectiveness of the treatments?

• Can I work while I'm undergoing therapy?

• Can I travel between treatments (short business or pleasure trips)?

• What test should be performed to determine if immunotherapy is right for me?

NOTES

CHAPTER 9: COMPLEMENTARY AND ALTERNATIVE THERAPIES

QUESTIONS TO ASK YOUR DOCTOR:

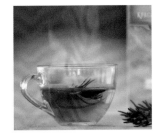

• What benefits can be expected from this therapy?

• Do the known benefits outweigh the risks?

• What side effects can be expected?

• Will the therapy interfere with conventional treatment?

• Will the therapy be covered by health insurance?

• Is medical cannabis a good option for me for managing pain or nausea?

NOTES

CHAPTER 10: CLINICAL TRIALS

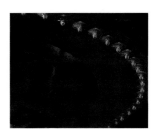

QUESTIONS TO ASK YOUR DOCTOR:

• Does being in a trial mean standard therapy has failed?

• Do you have other patients enrolled in trials?

• What trials are open in my area?

• How do I know the facility doing the study is reputable?

• What is involved in terms of tests, treatments, and additional time commitments?

• What results can be reasonably expected in my particular case?

• What are the currently accepted treatments and how do they compare to the trial?

• What would be my financial commitment?

• Will I need to be available for follow-up testing?

- What is the purpose of the study?

- How long will the trial last?

- Will results of the trial be available to me?

- What would be my financial commitment?

- Will I need to be available for follow-up testing?

- How will I know the experimental treatment is working?

CHAPTER 11: LIFE AFTER CANCER

QUESTIONS TO ASK YOUR DOCTOR:

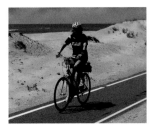

• Is there any point in quitting smoking now?

• What will replace smoking to help me handle stress?

• Can you suggest how I can change my habits so I can be healthier?

• What factors are the greatest risks to my cancer recurring?

• What is the best cancer follow-up schedule for me?

• What should I recommend to my relatives about lung cancer screening?

• How can I get involved so I help others afflicted by lung cancer?

NOTES

CHAPTER 12: ADVANCED CANCER

QUESTIONS TO ASK YOUR DOCTOR:

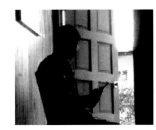

• What treatment options are available to me at this stage?

• Tell me about palliative care.

• Tell me about the hospice experience.

• Do I really need powerful drugs to control my pain?

• Is it OK if I take as little pain medication as possible?

• How long can I take narcotics for pain without getting addicted?

• Who can help me draw up documents such as advance directives, etc?

• Are there support groups my loved ones can join?

• How do I decide if it is time to stop treatment?

• What can I do to prepare for my death?

NOTES

CHAPTER 13: A GUIDE FOR YOUR PARTNER

QUESTIONS TO ASK YOUR DOCTOR:

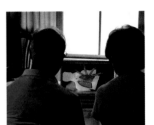

• Do you have any pamphlets, videos, or DVD's about lung cancer that we can take home and review?

• Is there a Resource Center or patient library in the facility where you practice?

• Who would you recommend we see for a second opinion?

• Can you put us in touch with others who you treated for this type of cancer, and with their partners?

• Will chemotherapy cause my hair to fall out?

NOTES

INDEX

My Healthcare Team

Nurse Navigator

_____
_____
_____

Primary

_____
_____
_____

Surgery

_____
_____
_____

Oncology

_____
_____
_____

Radiation Therapy

_____
_____
_____

Appointment Desk

_____
_____
_____

Nurse

_____
_____
_____

Nurse

_____
_____
_____

_____
_____
_____

_____
_____
_____